THE IDEAL BODY

YOU ARE NEVER TOO OLD TO GET ONE

By Jesus Antonio Caquias, MD

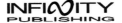

INFINITY PUBLISHING

Copyright © 2009, 2010 by Dr. Jesus Antonio Caquias

ISBN 0-7414-5873-X

Printed in the United States of America

Published March 2011

INFINITY PUBLISHING
1094 New DeHaven Street, Suite 100
West Conshohocken, PA 19428-2713
Toll-free (877) BUY BOOK
Local Phone (610) 941-9999
Fax (610) 941-9959
Info@buybooksontheweb.com
www.buybooksontheweb.com

DEDICATION

This book is dedicted to my children:
Brooke, Celenia, Miranda, Tomas and
Ninah

"Hear, my children,

the instruction of a father,

and give attention to know

understanding;

for I give you good doctrine:"

(Proverbs 4:1-2 NKJV)*

Contents

Recognition

I want to thank my wife Carmela, my son Tomas, my daughter Brooke, my brother Luis, my brother-in-law Seff Rodriguez, and my friends Richard Cantu, Juan Montoya, and Professor Amy Sierra Frazier for their comments and proofreading.

I want to thank Zito Kare, a great artist, my friend, and spiritual brother for the artwork that he so graciously provided.

"The LORD bless you and keep you;
The LORD make His face shine upon you,
And be gracious to you;
The LORD lift up His countenance upon you,
And give you peace."
(Numbers 6: 24-26 NKJV)*

Introduction

I was attending an Integrative Medicine class when the professor posed a question: "What is an ideal body?" This is an interesting question; I thought, but what actually constitutes an ideal body? Thus began my pondering as to whether an ideal body was within the bounds of possibilities. Can one have a reasonable expectation of achieving an ideal body as a result of specialized training, medical intervention, or care? Precisely, what does it mean to have an ideal body?

It is reasonable to postulate that an ideal body can only be quantified in relation to the environment in which it must adaptively survive. Obviously, if one were to survive like a fish underwater, one would have to meet a different set of criteria. The most extreme and ideal condition of being is to have the capacity and capability of existing with no ill effects to our conscious-ness in the multiplicity of environments that cosmic reality can bring to bear.

If such were possible, what would a body with such attributes be like? Would such a body be a "natural" or a "supernatral" body? If "supernatural," could we ever expect to achieve such and how? Does a person by dying pass into another realm of reality that can potentially give one such attributes?

Are we the end product of an evolutionary process or the beginning of one? Is it reasonably probable that the human body is merely a stepping-stone to a higher realm of consciousness and being for the purpose of achieving a very different existence, or must we be satisfied with it ending with death?

In what way do nature and the interaction of forces and God come to play a role in all of this? What are the determinants of an ideal body, and how is it that one comes about having one? Is it restricted to the physical body, or does the mind and morals play a role in its determination? Is it what is pleasing and sensuous to the eye? Or does it involve something more profound going beyond the flesh deep within the soul?

Is there evidence for an afterlife for which we must define "the ideal"? Or should we restrict our definition to the best criteria for surviving on this planet in our present environment and state of being?

The word "ideal" implies perfection, a concept existing only in the imagination. Or does it? Is there anyone presently, or has there been anyone in history, that has exhibited such attributes we can call ideal? I believe that there has been, and I will try to explain this in the ensuing narrative.

Chapter One

Energy or Matter

It was Einstein who theorized that matter could neither be created nor destroyed but only transformed. He theorized that matter and energy were two manifestations of the same substrate of reality comprised of the same components, matter being an extreme multidimensional organization of the energy, atomic, and subatomic particles contained therein.

In a brief paper which appeared in the German science magazine the *Annalen der Physics* in autumn of 1905, Einstein wrote; "If a body gives off the energy L in the form of radiation, its mass diminishes by L/c^2. The fact that the energy withdrawn from the body becomes energy of radiation evidently makes no difference. We are led to the more general conclusion that the mass of a body is a measure of its energy content; if the energy changes by L, the mass changes in the same sense by $L/9 \times 10^{20}$, the energy measured in ergs, and the mass in grams."[1]

All matter is comprised of atomic and subatomic particles. These particles contain immense amounts of energy, energy that we can cause to be released. The result has been that we have learned how to make matter into energy. We can now "split the atom." We do this when we initiate an atomic chain reaction like an atomic bomb. But we can also change matter into its constituent components. Burning, for example, is another form of this transformation. But is the better existence matter or energy?

Would an ideal body be one that would exist as a form of energy, such as what we call a spirit, that is, if we consider a spirit to exist as a form of energy? Or is an ideal body one that is made of matter such as flesh and blood?

Are we better as matter or as energy? Is there a means of measurement? If nothing can truly be destroyed but only changed and there is no real difference between matter and energy, can we say that one is better than the other? What is the difference that gives one more value?

There is, I believe, a difference which determines the superiority of existence. Whether you are an energy being or a material being, it would seem to me that the superior existence, assuming they both have self-consciousness, is determined by the abilities that the entity would have. The being with superior abilities would be the superior being.

Energy has no clear boundaries. The extent to which it reaches is outside of its control. Atomic and subatomic particles are influenced by the forces contained within them and those exerted from the outside. As energy becomes more organized, it takes on the qualities of matter. Forces from the outside have progessively less effect. Matter begins to set its own boundaries and takes on form.

Self-control is an aspect of superiority of all entities. Inanimate objects are less superior to animate living forms because they cannot exert influence beyond their boundaries. Higher life forms are superior to lower life forms by the mere fact that they are able to control the lower life forms. By life forms, I am referring to organisms that are able to reproduce.

Spiritual beings are assumed to be superior because they are believed to have supernatural abilities beyond those of natural beings. This is demonstrated in much literature concerning spiritual beings.

A body capable of self-determination, having the power of reason and emotion, able to choose and to act, to accept or give direction, to transcend its own boundaries or change its form, and is able to sustain itself, would constitute an ideal body.

In a limited way, we, as human beings, have some of these abilities. We possess free will. We exert control over our surroundings. We decide. We give direction. But we cannot change our form or transcend our boundaries, and we are not self-sustaining.

A higher being, one that can transcend its boundaries, is able to create, change its form, and sustain life, we call God. The ideal body would be able to transcend its boundaries, change its form, sustain, and control its own self, thus have some Godlike attributes.

Accepting its limitations, the human body is still an incredible creation. The complexities of our different organ systems form a marvelous constellation – a constellation as incredible as those of the very universe – having billions of tiny organisms - units called cells, working together to maintain its form and function. Truly, it is an incredible creation.

Like tiny soldiers, each cell mans its post carrying out its duties to the very death. Each cell is preprogrammed to deal with what could naturally come against it. Yet, not alone, each cell is assisted by other cells, some from a significant distance away - forming an intricate relational work force that functions to maintain the body in a very precise manner.

Still, the human body is far from ideal. It must rely on a continuous supply of an external energy supply — a food source. It is delicate, vulnerable to numerous environmental attacks. It must also periodically rest, or it will suffer negative health consequences. Such attributes demonstrate the limitations of the human body.

We were made to be dependent on each other and our environment. Presently, we do not have a full understanding of all of the forces and environmental variables upon which our existence depends.

While our body may be adequate for our present environment, it is far from ideal! When one considers the amount of energy the human body must expend to keep going and how vulnerable it is in comparison to other creatures in our world, one is struck by the many things one can think of adding to make the human body ideal. This has given rise to the many concepts of "superheroes" we have seen depicted on television and various magazines and newspapers.

Chapter 1

1. It was Einstein who theorized that matter can neither be created nor destroyed but only _____.

2. All matter is comprised of _____ and _____ particles.

3. If nothing can truly be destroyed but only changed and there is no real _____ between matter and energy, can we say that one is better than the other?

4. Like tiny soldiers, each cell serves at its post carrying out its duties to the very _____.

5. We were made to be _____ on each other and on our environment.

6. While our body may be adequate for our present environment, it is far from _____!

Answers: transformed, atomic, subatomic, difference, death, dependent, ideal

Chapter Two

Energy Acquisition

Do you ever wonder what would make an ideal digestive system? Why do we need to eat such varieties of foods or drink water? Why is it that an animal like a kangaroo rat can get all its water from what it eats and we have to be constantly drinking water?

Our digestive system leaves much to be desired. Yes, it provides a means for us to acquire our nutrient needs. But the resultant waste is great. Why isn't our body more efficient? Why do we have to get oxygen through breathing? Why are we not able to get all of our nutrition and energy requirements from the air we breathe, from the water, or just from the food we take in? The various functions have to work together to provide us with what we need for energy and to sustain ourselves.

If there is energy all around us, why can we not assimilate this energy and use it for our own purposes? Why do we produce so much waste? It does not seem that our gastrointestinal system is very efficient. There are tens of thousands of waste-treatment plants around the world that can attest to that!

An ideal gastrointestinal system would be one hundred percent efficient. An ideal body in my opinion would be one that would not even need to eat. It would be able to assimilate its energy from its surroundings, from the air or from the environment it lives in and yet could eat and not form any waste because it could digest and use up all substances completely.

It would not even have to breathe. It would get all it needs for energy from the energy sources around it. This may sound pretty incredible, but think about it. Do we not spend a lot of time simply trying to keep this body going? It is far from ideal.

Atoms never stop moving. Yet, they do not eat. Why should we? After all, are we not made of the same components? Why, then, are we unable to get charged up by the exchange of electrons like the atoms we are composed of? If energy is indestructible and only subject to change, should we not be able to get our energy requirements from our surroundings?

If we had an ideal body, we would possess such qualities as those of atomic particles. This may sound absurd to some, but our bodies are comprised of the same atomic particles and we should, therefore, ideally have the same qualities. We were not, for whatever reason, designed to have such qualities.

We, like nearly everything around us, are doomed to decay. We leave only a trace of our existence in the genes of our descendants. Still, is this the ideal? Is immortality not better? Or is immortality defined by the passage of traits we pass on to our progeny?

Certainly, one could appreciate the world's situation if everyone who was ever born were alive today. As vulnerable as our bodies are to the environment that we live in, could we still survive? Would we be able to maintain life in a world with limited food supply and limited space?

We would need a different world or a different body, an ideal body!

If we could survive by assimilating needed energy from the bombardment of the countless of atoms around us, the food problem would not exist. But could we say that this would be the ideal?

Does death provide a means for continued life? Is the present the ideal in this current world? Or are we on a journey which culminates or begins with death? Is death the end? Or is it the beginning?

Considering what is ideal, one must consider the suitability of the environment which the body must inhabit. If we are to live only off the land, reproduce, and die, then our bodies may be said to be adequate yet still far from ideal.

Our waste production is too great to consider our bodies even efficient in this current world. Our food requirements and waste production forces us to devise collective solutions. It is nearly impossible for an individual to live comfortably alone. We are interdependent beings. We impact each other intentionally and unintentionally for benefit and at times in a detrimental manner.

Our survival depends on our ability to work collectively to solve the problems our existence creates. Whether one believes this to be a product of design or part of an evolutionary process, it is still far from the ideal.

Chapter 2

1. If there is energy all around us, why can we not _____ this energy and use it for our own purposes?

2. An ideal gastrointestinal system would be one that would be _____ percent efficient.

3. Why are we not able to get all of our nutrition and _____ requirements from the air we breathe, from the water, or just from the food we take in?

4. We, like nearly everything around us, are doomed to _____.

5. We leave only a trace of our existence in the _____ of our descendants.

6. Our survival depends on our ability to work _____ to solve the problems our existence creates.

Answers: assimilate, one hundred, energy, decay, genes, collectively

Chapter Three

Avoiding Destruction

It seems we are constantly struggling to survive. Our body is constantly under attack. We struggle against the balance of nature. Unfortunately, decay is an undeniable fact and a necessary aspect of our existence.

The very microorganisms that make life possible by destroying our waste are the same organisms that could potentially make life impossible for us. An ideal body would be one that would not be vulnerable to destruction by microorganisms such as those that could now destroy us.

Our immune system is incredibly complicated. We have cells preprogrammed to identify and destroy foreign invaders that may enter our body. There are millions of different receptor sites on our immune cells for the purpose of recognizing and inciting defense reactions that result in the elimination and destruction of the foreign invader.

Our immune cells, like many of the other cells in our body, have extraordinary sensory perception. Bioenergetic signaling between cells provides an incredible communication system, one that rivals the world's communication and Internet network. Immune cells talk to one another and to other cells through receptor signaling substances by way of receptor protein sites on their surfaces.

We know from the evolution of our own communi-cation network that we can signal electronically without hard wires by way of various electronic frequencies.

Proteins and other chemically charged substances act like the hard wires in our communication network. The ideal would be if our cells were capable of sending electronic frequencies, capable of communicating with other cells much like our wireless computers.

Ideal body cells would be capable of discharging fre-quencies that would serve to protect us from foreign invaders or raise an impregnable barrier that would neutralize such invasion by some energetic means.

In science fiction, we conjure up such protection as force fields, impregnable barriers to invasion. But in real life, such protection would be impractical. Aside from needing protection from destructive organisms, we are beings that thrive on relationships.

Life would not be enjoyable or even livable without our ability to relate to other human beings or to our environment. We are social beings. Life and beauty would have no significance without our ability to share them. Generally, anyone who fails to seek such interactions is considered not to be in their right mind and categorized as being ill.

An ideal immune system is one that would not fall prey to an invading microorganism. The body would in some way repel or neutralize the potential invader. However, attacking and breaking down biological forms is necessary in a world where all things must be recycled.

Decomposition or putrefaction is a process by which our world is cleaned up. Without the process of decay, we could not have life. The millions upon millions of organisms dedicated to cleaning up our environment are incredible. They are a necessary aspect of our existence.

Imagine what the world would be like if all life forms of yesteryears were still around today. Our world was made to regenerate its life forms in a perfectly balanced ecosystem.

For example, we have in our world millions of insects, most of which we cannot even see. These insects not only function to consume the bigger components that need to be destroyed but also act as transport vehicles for the smaller microorganisms that deal with decay at the microscopic level.

As unappealing as some of these insects may appear to be to us, they were crafted as such for their own survival and for their own very special function. Their special function is not even apparent to most people, that is, to bring in the initiators of decay, the microorganism – or what we call germs – that decompose the waste other organisms produce, in turn making food for their transporting host.

The dung beetle is one example. Anyone who has ever disturbed a dung pile that has been on the ground for a few days would find it infested with these beetles. The beetles also bring microorganisms which assist them in obtaining their meal. These creatures have been designed specifically for such a purpose, as are many of the other insects in the world which seem to have specialized and peculiar functions. Another very well recognized insect that functions as such is the common housefly.

Our own intestinal bacterial flora acts in this way. They eat our waste and produce additional food for us. When we have bacteria that do not produce nutrients but instead produce toxins, we have disease. We begin to decay. The concept of taking probiotics, or beneficial bacteria, is based on helping our body improve our health and avoid disease.

Overall, ecological communities in the world hang in a delicate balance, between living and dying, nourishment and decay, operating for the maintenance of some great design in a phenomenal ecological balance.

The function and the reason for the sheer number of insects are readily apparent; they have an immense job to do. One thing that has always amazed me is how some of these creatures were made to appear. Their features are truly amazing. Why were they designed to parallel the appearance of other species in the animal kingdom? Was this merely an evolutionary coincidence or the sign of a common creator?

Take the rhinoceros beetle for example. Isn't it interesting that such an insect would exist? This is not the only insect with a parallel appearance. Even some microorganisms are very similar to the minute cells we are composed of. Is this proof of evolution or the sign of a common creator God?

From looking at the incredible life forms, one can only conclude that if they were created by some intelligent being the being obviously loves to create. This creator deliberately made creatures that were not only fascinating but in many ways also resemble different species. Is this coincidental, or is the creator God providing us with evidence of His existence?

Can we conclude that since the rhinoceros beetle and the rhinoceros have similar appearances that they must have derived from a common ancestor? Is that not what we have done by comparing a cell from our body to a single cell organism and concluding that we must have started as a single cell organism? The comparison and conclusions are totally ridiculous.

In art, we see patterns of structure and style that readily identify the artist. Is this the same thing that we are seeing in nature? Each one of us must arrive at our own conclusion. If there is a creator God, we must also consider what He would do for our refusal to give Him recognition.

The genome or "genetic map" for example, is remarkably similar in most species, even in prehistotic creatures. Yet it codes for very dissimilar species. Genes are turned off or are not switched on, making for very different appearing species. This is like finding the paint, or medium, or style, used by a particular artist. While this would help us identify the artist, in real life, we instead ridicule Him, saying, "You could not have done this; it just happened by itself"!

Do not artists become indignant when we fail to give them credit for their art work? Think how much more incensed the creator, who makes possible our existence, would be for our failure to acknowledge Him?

When archeologists come across complex unnatural formations, they conclude that they represent the creation of some ancient culture. They begin to look for connections with other cultures. They do not begin to look at how such things could have come about by themselves. They readily understand that some intelligent being had to have made it.

Complex design is a sign of intelligent creation and speaks to the existence of an intelligent creator.

Yet, in nature, those, with the preconceived notion that there is not a God, immediately look at evolution and disregard the possibility of intelligent design by a creator God. The vast similarities of design and the interdependency of so many millions of life forms should lead one to the conclusion that an intelligent being had to be involved in creation. Such infinite coincidences without intelligent intervention are not possible.

Chapter 3

1. We struggle against the balance of nature. Unfortunately, _____ is an undeniable fact and a _____ aspect of our existence.

2. An ideal body would be one that would not be _____ to _____ by microorganisms such as those that could now destroy us.

3. We have cells _____ to identify and destroy foreign invaders that could enter our bodies.

4. When we have bacteria that do not produce nutrients but instead produce toxins, we have _____.

5. In art, we see patterns of structure and style that readily identify the _____.

6. The vast similarities of design and the _____ of so many millions of life forms should lead one to the conclusion that an intelligent being had to be involved in creation.

Answers: decay, necessary, vulnerable, destruction, preprogrammed, disease, artist, interdependency

Chapter Four

By Design or by Chance

In science, a repetition of sound or complex unnatural construction implies a creative source. For example, consider the monitoring of ionic and radio waves from outer space for signs of communications from intelligent beings. The Earth is constantly hit with scattered radio waves. How would we recognize a message coming from an intelligent being? By their repetition! Monitoring radio waves and targeting consistent repetitive patterns is the method used to distinguish intelligent intent from random scattered radio waves. Like the messages that we send out, we would expect that the messages that we receive would be organized and repetitious.

Turn the monitors around toward earth. Is there not repetition in everything around us, even within us? Does a commonality of creation reveal a common creator? Do we not build on what we know when we work on a project? If such is the case, can there be a purposeful plan behind the creation of man and the universe? Should we instead accept the universe as coming into being by chance and for no reason?

If there is no designer and no plan, does all that there is end when death comes? Are we to judge the ideal within the constraints of a life and death existence? Or is there a bigger plan that must be taken into account?

If creation came about simply by a common process in which all things evolved, how was the process established and why? If some creator set up the process, why set up such an inefficient and combersome system? A system that functions by mere accidental events does not need a god. To think that God would use such a system is foolish.

Certainly, if there were such a creator who could establish the forces that would bring about and protect His creation, that creator would have sufficient power to bring such things about in an instant, in the blink of an eye.

For life to come about and for it to be sustained, even simple life forms require a myriad of exact circumstances. These exact circumstances would be impossible, except they were pre-established by some intelligent guiding force before life appeared.

The exact circumstances and the sustaining forces required for life to thrive are precise and unchangeable. The delicate balance of chemistry, correct temperatures, and exact forces, (gravitational, electromagnetic, nuclear, and otherwise) have to be exactly as they are for life to exist, let alone evolve. These are, in addition to such factors as the orbits of the earth and moon, the earth's tilt, the issues of pressure, atmospheric composition and filtering of surface radiation, water supply, and numerous other requirements, needed for life to thrive.

If the atomic weghts of the subatomic particles were not as they are, then hydrogen could not form, and we would not have a sun, the stars, or the cosmos as we know it. The precision, with which the corresponding forces and laws adhere, can be computed to within a range of multiple decimal points.

The marvelous creation, the precision with which everything has come into existence, points to a deliberate and well-engineered plan. The resulting product must also be precise and calculated for some awe-inspiring purpose. To believe that all these things occurred by chance is absurd.

Such precision would require a creator with infinite knowledge of all requisite components for life as we know it. Only a God of precision could have designed us and the universe that we live in. With the many precise variables that are required, none of this could have occurred by chance.

The genesis of life is not as simple as evolutionists would have us believe. Many of the proteins required for life are made up of thousands of amino acids that have to be sequenced in a specific manner for proper function so as to sustain life. These proteins must interact with other proteins in a precise and constructive manner, or the organism would not be viable.

For this purpose, God created the DNA, an authoritarian molecule which by switching and various other controls commands for speciation and a billion of other variables. This is God's tool for creation. A precision instrument had to have been deliberately designed for such purpose and which could not have come about by chance in a trillion years due to its vastly complex nature. That we should come across it and deny that it had to have been divinely created is worthy of retribution.

A molecular geneticist with knowledge of the complexities involved in gene transfer would not deny the prerequisite knowledge and detail that is involved in transferring a single gene. To determine that genetic engineering for the purpose of speciation could occur sponataneously is to say that complex construction can come about without intellectual intervention.

Many thousands of interactions have to be precisely arranged. The interactions require multiple gene changes that must occur simultaneously for the genetic coding to produce functional proteins that will contribute to the viability of the organism.

Take striated muscle for example. Connectin or titin is the largest known protein containing over thirty-four thousand amino acids. Not only does the large number of amino acids require proper sequencing, but the amino acids must also interact and connect in a precise manner. The protein must interact with multiple muscle sarcomere proteins; rely on calcium released from calcium channels, and ATP produced by mitochondria for proper function. This is many times more complicated than most precise instruments produced by man.

How many directional messages are contained in one DNA strand? The numbers are staggering, yet each nucleotide is arranged in a very precise manner. Can we truly say such precision, organization, and direction can occur of itself? Not in our universe!

Darwin, in his "ORIGIN OF THE SPECIES" advised his followers, "If it could be demonstrated that any complex organ existed which could not possibly have been formed by numerous, successive, slight modifications, my theory would absolutely break down."[2] This statement and the complexities demonstrated in living forms makes creation through evolution according to Darwin impossible.

That we can take nucleotides and splice them into different sites and create variations within a species does not prove creation through evolution. Species diversity occurs frequently in nature and accounts for the variations within species not for their creation. Creation requires many more complex and precision placement of specific nucleotides and switches to form a new species. Creation of new species entails changes that would require vast knowledge and understanding that is impossible by random chance.

Darwin had sufficient intelligence and sincerety to know that the variations he was observing in species could not explain complex changes that were as yet poorly understood. Our present understanding of the complexities of our genes and immense work and understanding needed to engineer a simple variation should make us conclude that such complex changes could not occur without intelligent design.

Contrary to the theory of evolution, even the simplest life forms are very complex. Work with the smallest known genome that of Mycoplasma genitalium, a parasitic bacterium that lives in the epithelium of the respiratory and genital tract of primates, demonstrates the presence of at least 250 to 350 gene products which have been documented. [3,4] Biophysicist Hubert Yockey calculated the probability of spontaneously forming a single gene product as one chance in 10 to the 75th power[5]. If the universe were 15 billion years old, less than one trillionth of the time has passed of what is needed to make one of the 250 to 350 gene products necessary for the Mycoplasma genitalium bacterium, [6,7] a drop in the ocean of time needed to form only one gene product.

Biomolecular sciences and genetics have permitted us to understand certain complexities of nature. However, we continue with the belief that it all came about through evolution. Darwin understood that evolution could not create complex organs and we now know that even a single cell has thousands of complex organelles.

The study of the human genome has further bolstered the divine creation doctrine by demonstrating that current humans are the probable descendants of a single pair of individuals.

There have been multiple studies on the nucleotide base pair segments of the Y chromosome in ethnically diverse groups of men. The studies have consistantly demonstrated that the men all descended from one man that lived less then 270,000 years ago.[8]

Mitochondria are found in the cytoplasma of the cell and are derived from the mother. Mitochondrial DNA analysis in ethnically diverse groups of people has demonstrated that all humans are descendants of one woman living less than 250,000 years ago.

In 1993 at the meeting of the American Association for the Advancement of Science Maryellen Ruvolo from Harvard University, researchers presented data that used DNA sequencing rather than restriction analysis to study part of the cytochrome oxidase genome and found that it affirmed the findings of current humans being descendants of one woman living less than 200,000 years ago.[9]

Gorillas, orangutans, and chimpanzees show large variations in the Y chromsome when compared to man but little variation among each other. If man had descended from such primates, less variation would have been found between primates and man.[10] The findings refuted the expectation that these primates were from the distant past and affirmed that they must be from recent origins as are the humans.

Single-organism evolution is not only extremely complex, but also if they are to reproduce, such species must have a companion that must evolve in the exact manner at the same approximate time. They then have to come in intimate contact for reproduction to be even possible.

Since there are millions of species that reproduce sexually, they, therefore, must have comparable companions. The companions must also evolve in the exact manner during the same time period and in the same vicinity as they do. The intricately complex evolutionary process must have occurred billions of times to have brought about the millions of creatures that have existed on the planet since the existence of sexually reproducing and co-dependent species.

Evolutionists expect us not only to believe that in evolution spontaneous chemical reactions formed life but that co-evolution, the spontaneous creation of interdependent life forms, also occurred spontaneously and simultaneously since such forms could not survive without the other.

Many life forms depend on other life forms. They have obligate symbiotic relationships without which neither species could survive. These creatures would have had to have evolved simultaneously since each depends on the other for their existance.

This involves plants that require pollinating insects, specific fungus that only grow on the decaying bodies of certain insects and obligate parasites which require a specific host to survive. There are millions of such examples.

Our best example of this complex interdependence is the evolution of the male and female of the species. One without the other could not make for a continuance of the species. This involves separate evolutionary processes where one develops into a male and the other into a female by separate evolutionary means. The argument that one sex evolved into both sexes denies the fossil record. Both the male and the female are needed to produce an offspring.

Every sexual creature has the same requirement. Each has to evolve into the counterpart of the other. This has to occur at or around the same time period within an area where they would have a high likelihood of having contact. This is absolutely necessary for the pair to reproduce and permit the species to continue.

Are we to accept that a series of accidents could result in precision construction, a process that is contrary to every working in nature? The vast majority of spontaneous genetic changes are destructive not constructive. The purposeful hand of a creator is needed.

The likelihood of creation happening on its own and the intricately complex processes that must occur simultaneously is not possible even in the most favorable of conditions. Yet, we are expected to believe that it could occur in a hostile and destructive environment.

This is like expecting to win the lottery each and every time for the next hundred years. Only a fool would believe that such complex processes could occur by chance,

"The fool says in his heart, 'There is no God.' They are corrupt, their deeds are vile; there is no one who does well." (Psalms 14:1 NKJV)* God looks down on us and says: "Have I not given you a brain, why do you refuse to use it?"

Complex creatures require intricately complex interacting modifications which had to have developed at the same time, or the species could not survive. When we talk about a complex organism evolving, we are not simply speaking about a single chance occurrence every so many millions of years. We are speaking about multiple changes, and at times thousands of changes, or millions of changes occurring all at once.

Since a single change may require thousands of modifications, such creatures would not survive with single modifications one at a time due to their complex interdependent nature.

Biologists hypothesize that such gradual changes can occur over time, a process called gradualism. They use gradualism to explain the gradual changes seen over time in the fossil record. Rapid change, occurring in a short time and being maintained for a long period of time, is called punctuated equilibrium. However, the differences could be explained by diversity among the species brought about by environmental pressures or could represent a related species of the same family.

However we look at it, the protein coding and the required interactions with the other proteins and chemistry of the species is a great deal more complex than the phenotypic or visible changes that we see in the organism. It is like getting a new sofa in a home that is already cluttered with furniture. The other furniture would have to be moved to make room for the new sofa. Even the smallest change would have multiple ramifications.

Each component of a cell is like a microscopic machine working in perfect harmony with other components in the cell and with distant cells through their interactive proteins to sustain the cell and maintain its function. It is not as simple as evolutionists would have us believe. There has not been any scientific explanation on how these exceedingly complex systems could have evolved because there is no way to explain them adequately. They just had to come into being suddenly. That is, they had to have been created suddenly as they are.

To expect people to accept that evolution by random natural selection led to speciation is to accept that chance has knowledge and direction. Genetisists are now calling diversity "evolution" to make evolution a more acceptable concept. Diversity represents species variation which is an adaptive mechanism for survival. Creating a new trait in a species in the laboratory through gene transfer does not prove that random natural selection led to speciation as many claim. They ignore all that they had to do to create the variant. What they have proven is that it takes a creator to create even a small variant in an organism as they have done.

Their real goal is to firm up the belief in evolution so as to bolster their funding. They better than most understand the complexities involved and how difficult and precise this work has to be. For a totally new species, the amount of work and required manipulation and knowledge is much more than that of introducing a simple trait. That is exactly why in nature it would be impossible without a creator.

Could the great deceiver be behind this? Could we have bought a bill of goods whose only purpose is to lead us down a path of destruction? Does the philosophy of survival of the fittest actually serve man? Evolutionists say that it does. But does it really? Speciation is not a simple random process as many would misrepresent it to be. It is much more complex, involving many different interactions, more than most people can even imagine.

Take the giraffe for instance. If the cardiovascular system adaptations had not developed simultaneously with their long necks, they could not survive. On raising its head for the very first time, it would suffer a stroke and die. These vastly complex adaptations have to evolve simultaneously, and at the same time, the opposite sex of the species has to undergo these same adaptations.

Can anyone truly believe that such a multitude of precise changes could occur by chance without some direction from the outside? Are we so untrue to ourselves that we can believe that these things could occur on their own without an intelligent designer?

Every organism appears to have a function in the maintenance, destruction, and rebuilding processes of our planet and in God's plan. Even organisms that survive in extreme hostile environments such as extremophiles may have some function. That they were designed for such a purpose falls within the doctrine of creation by God. As is written *"The heavens declare the glory of God; and the firmament shows His handiwork." (Psalm 19:1 NKJV)*

Extremeophiles defy evolution. Extreme enzymes require an extreme environment and an intact organism for their production. The organism requires the extreme enzyme for their survival and proliferation. These had to come together at the same time. With man learning how to manufacture some of these enzymes, man proves a creator is required for their origination whether it be on earth or any extraterrestrial body. How could an organism evolve and thrive in such hostile environments if they had not been designed for such in the first place? I would not be surprised to hear of extremeophile organisms in more extreme places or even on distant planets. These extremeophile organisms may play a role in the ecological fabric of the universe, an understanding we have not yet attained.

Those of us who accept that we and everything in the universe are the creation of an all knowing God do not have to ponder how it came about. We cannot see Him. But there is a world of evidence that He exists and we see it in everything around us. He spoke it into existence, and it came into being. Afterwards, He sat back so that His great plan could play itself out, as you will read in the following pages.

There is a world that we see that is material and a world that we do not see that is beyond the senses. In fact, there is more that we do not see than what we can see. Additionally, there is much to suggest that we hang in a delicate balance between what we see and what we cannot see.

As our spirituality becomes more in tune with the spiritual, we begin to appreciate that there is something more than that which we can comprehend. There is another dimension that seems to touch our lives mysteriously. We all experience it at one time or another. That experience makes us ask the question: Is there a God?

I hate to think that life and death is all that there is, that it all ends when we die. Think of it. If we were to have an ideal body, would death threaten us? To have to face death is not to be ideal. But is there a continuum, a crossover, whereby we go from this material world with all of its imperfections to the energetic or spiritual world that cannot be destroyed? Is there a reason for our existence? Are we the result of a great plan? And is there any evidence for such a plan?

Einstein's theory of relativity is one that has always intrigued me. The thought that time could stand still is incredible. Simply stated, time stops when we move at the speed of light. This is a profound mathematical concept with equally profound philosophical as well as religious implications. Just think about it; time ceases, time stands still when you move at the speed of light. How could this be? Is not time a relative event, a measure of one interval to the next? How is it that it could stop? It is unbelievable, but yet it has been demonstrated to be true.

The theory of relativity implies that there is no such thing as time for the atomic and subatomic particles that make up this universe, or even still, that constitutes our own makeup. Yet, Einstein's theory has been proven again and again. As we have undertaken space travel, we have had to take into account the effect that speed has on time.

How about energetic beings? Are they outside the constraints of time? God dwells in His own chosen realm where time has no utility. In essence, there is no such thing as time for God. This concept has been put forth since the beginning of recorded history. Through his mathematical theorizing, Einstein was able to ascertain in a stuctured fashion a concept long held as a requisite for God's divinity, this concept, however, until Einstein's theory was without validity.

Man's concept of creation through evolution is like trying to unscramble scrambled eggs. The question becomes — given the complexity of the task and the limitation of available methods and means — would our attempt at unscrambling the scrambled egg result in a true and correct facsimile of the real egg? One can certainly accept whatever the unscrambling reveals, but would it be correct?

That is exactly what we have done with evolution. In the end, it comes down to whatever one wants to believe, hoping, of course, that the belief is not wrong. I personally would choose that belief which carries with it the lesser of the consequences and provides the greatest reward.

If the theory of relativity is true, then how long is one day for God? How much of man's time is there in one of God's days? How much can God do in one day where time does not exist?

Are we so knowledgeable that we can make such a determination, or must we simply accept what He tells us? If we refuse to accept the details that He has chosen to give us, then are we ready to accept the consequences?

Denial will not rid you of the consequences that He may choose to impose upon you, and what's more, you will have no excuse. The evidence abounds; your refusal to accept it will not change that.

How much can we put into a point the size of a period on this page? Imagine that we could compress everything so tightly that everything in the universe would fit into a point the size of a period. That is how scientists say it was before the "big bang." Everything started at a point the size of a period on this page. Can you believe it?

Is it easier to believe that we could get everything in the universe into a point the size of a period than that God did it by simply speaking it into being? The point is that both are difficult concepts to accept. Yet most will readily accept the period concept and not accept the God concept because to do so would impose accountability on the individual.

If the God concept is a true concept, denying it will not remove any consequences of its denial. The period concept calls to question how it all came about, whom or what caused it. That everything in the universe could fit into a point the size of a period is beyond the imagination. It is supernatural, and only a supernatural being could bring this about. That being is God.

A supernatural being that could bring about the big bang would not have time or distance limitations as such an individual would be beyond the atomic, beyond the natural. He could be wherever He wants, whenever He wants without restriction, and even simultaneously in as many places as He wants.

Likewise, can we measure an instant in God's timing when time does not exist? Time and distance are relative terms for the natural world in which we live. They are not applicable in the supernatural.

Can we measure a spiritual concept with a natural device and consider it valid? Scripture states, *"God is Spirit, and those who worship Him must worship in spirit and truth." (John 4:24 NKJV)**

That distance has no relevancy to God is demonstrated by the big bang theory itself, as small as a period on this page, or as spectacular as the universe, God covers all of them. Like a force field that traverses all things, that is God.

The universe is said to be expanding, the result of the big bang explosion. Yet scripture declares that God Himself expanded the universe. *"It is He who sits above the circle of the earth, And its inhabitants are like grasshoppers, Who stretches out the heavens like a curtain, And spreads them out like a tent to dwell in."(Isaiah 40:22 NKJV)*

Notice that the Bible declared that the earth was round thousands of years before it was actually discovered to be round. This could have only been divinely revealed by a supernatural God.

All of this may sound irrational to some, but man has been trying to measure the supernatural by natural means for as long as unbelief has been around. It seems respectable to arrive at wild conclusions in the natural but unacceptable to do so in the supernatural. Yet arriving at wild conclusions in the supernatural is more logical since the supernatural has no limitations. To place natural limits of measurements on the supernatural makes no sense. It shows how foolish our thinking is.

Take for example a 30-year-old person traveling through a hypothetical space-time wormhole 50 years into the future. To the people on the other side, this individual would be 80 years old, but to the individual, he would still only be 30 years old. Their assessment would make no sense. Likewise, it is the same for God for whom no time or distance exists. Man's assessment of the supernatural makes no sense. The supernatural cannot be measured by natural means. It can only be accepted as what it is: supernatural!

God can be standing somewhere in the United States and take one step east and be in China. Or, conversely, He could take one step south and be at the South Pole. Would our physical measurements about how far God traveled or how long God took to get there have any relevance or any truth?

The God of Abraham, Isaac, and Jacob, the Father God of Jesus the Christ, the Messiah, the Anointed One, is not limited by physical laws. He can still the wind, calm the raging sea, walk on water, or make physical time stop. He is not limited by nature. He is the God of nature, the ruler of the universe! He is not limited by our natural laws. He makes the laws do whatever He wants.

God loves to create. One only need look at the wonderful and numerous marvels of His creation to know that God loves to create. He loves life, and color, and beauty, and splendor. He is not an egotist that He should want man solely to be constantly worshiping Him. He wants man to enjoy what He loves. God has made man so that by their trials and tribulations He could create perfect beings, divine like Himself for His holy kingdom, the epitome of His creation.

Religious leaders who claim to represent the supernatural creator God of the Bible and buy into the natural evolutionary explanation of creation that consider the Genesis story a myth fail to understand the nature of God. Their devotion is to another god and not to the supernatural creator God of the Bible.

We cannot accept much of what is in the Judeo Christian Bible if we do not accept the supernatural nature of God. And if we accept that God is supernatural and is able to perform immeasurable supernatural feats, we cannot accept man's attempt to explain the feats by natural means.

All creation reveals a great design with incredible mathematical relationships. Einstein's theories and mathematical calculations prove this to be a fact. These mathematical relationships are extremely precise and could not occur by chance but only by purposeful design.

While we have trouble accepting that there are moral absolutes for behavior, the fact is that everything in the universe must obey absolute mathematical laws of relationships or the universe could not exist.

Forces in nature are precise and not arbitrary. From the pull of gravity to the forces that keep atoms together, all must be precisely what they are or there would not be a universe as we know it.

The interesting thing about it is that it all seems to have been made to make our existence possible. This sounds incredible. Could we be that important? Or is there another reason for it? Does God have a plan, and is He building something that is more important than anything that He has done before? It certainly seems like it!

The established consensus among those that deny divine design is that all creatures evolved from less complex creatures which evolved from single-cell organisms that evolved by chance from the interaction of various chemicals. A divine designer is not needed.

Even some religious leaders accept such arguments as a possible method used by the creator. If such were the case, what kind of a god would that be? You cannot call such an entity a god. Or can God be limited by nature and still be God?

What kind of a creator would God be if he had only to stand by while creation just happened? He would not be much of a God, for such a God would Himself be subject to nature.

Evolutionists say that because creation through evolution is so slow and takes vast time spans to create minute changes, we can never prove or disprove it. That is an interesting thought. But it has been reported that we are losing thousands of species on a daily basis. Millions of species have already disappeared.

The process in place is destructive, not constructive. How is it that creation through evolution could be taking place? If the adaptive forces of creation through evolution were truly at work, then species would continue to form and their numbers would increase, not decrease. Why have so many disappeared?

I can recall my genetics class assignment at The Brooklyn Center of Long Island University while working on my bachelor's degree. We took tiny fruit flies known by their scientific name as Drosophilae and exposed them to different mutation-causing agents such as x-rays, ultraviolet light, and various chemicals. This resulted in some fruit flies with curly wings, some with white eyes, and others with various mutations. Yet, as interesting as these induced mutations were, I never saw or heard of a house fly come about as a result of these experiments.

We have identified nearly all variants, and despite their trait, they were still considered the same species. These days, the tiny fruit fly is being subjected to gene transfer from other species, making for additional variants. These variants are being called "new species," though they differ only by the trait given to them by the gene transfer. This is being celebrated as proof of creation through evolution, but is it really, or is there deception in this representation? Does not creation through evolution require speciation by natural selection? Is not the geneticist acting as God? Are they not actually proving that speciation requires a creator, that is, if we can call the new variant a new species?

These experiments demonstrate diversity within the species, different variations that can occur in a species brought on by environmental pressures. Some call this micro-evolution which is a misnomer since the species remains the same and the variant features can be bred out.

The experiments were very interesting. However, in thousands of universities around the world, for over eighty years, the same experiments have been conducted. Not one has reported the development of a new and different species of fly in these experiments.

The exposure to mutation-causing agents all these many years would be equivalent to millions of years of exposure in the wild. Yet not one new and different species of fly has been created. Has creation through evolution been disproven inadvertently in our genetics laboratories?

Can we accept that perhaps there is no such thing as creation through evolution and that we are in fact devolving instead of evolving? Is all that there is, and all that there has been, actually the work of a great creator who stopped creating new creatures for some reason and left us on our own for some great purpose?

Creationists claim evolution cannot occur since it violates the first and second laws of thermodynamics, that is, that everything left to its own breaks down, that energy is dispersed, that entropy is increased. This is true of everything in the universe. But could not the Creator make an exception for living forms, as perhaps only He could? But why — if He could just speak it and there it is — why would He just let it happen?

Would a God that could create the elements and the universe need a process? And is the process of creating the planets, the stars, and everything that is found in the constellations any more difficult than creating life? Would He be God if He could not create life?

Some say that the healing of the body violates the laws of thermodynamics. But does it? Does not healing require genetic instruction, the very instructions that are encoded in the genes? Healing is not spontaneous but occurs under genetic direction and with the induction of the various chemical reactions initiated after an injury.

Species variation, or diversity, is not a valid argument for creation or for speciation by natural selection. Variations are required for species survival, and the variant code already exists in the species. Adaptation is a requirement for maintenance of life. Being able to adapt to changes in one's environment is as important as being able to reproduce.

Without species diversity, adaptation and survival would not be possible in a changing environment. However, it does not prove creation. Speciation requires much more complex changes beyond species diversity. Truly, new species would not be able to interbreed and produce progeny.

With diversity, the genetic code already exists in the species. It simply needs the environmental pressures to be expressed. With the creation of a new and different species, a new genetic code must form and not just a single code, but multiple, beneficial, and supportive codes must occur spontaneously and simultaneously in the co-dependent organism to effect a viable genetic change.

I cannot accept evolution as the means for creation since there is no evidence that complex beneficial changes can occur spontaneously and simultaneously in their co-dependent partner, as must of necessity have occurred during creation. I, therefore, must believe that there is a supernatural creator God who can speak all things into existence and who has done so for His divine plan and purpose!

Chapter 4

1. Like the messages that we send out, we would expect that the messages that we would receive would be organized and _____.

2. Many of the proteins required for life are made up of thousands of _____ that have to be sequenced in a specific manner for proper function and maintenance of life.

3. Each component of a cell is like a microscopic machine working in perfect _____ with other components in the cell and in distant cells through their interactive proteins to sustain the cell and maintain its function for the organism.

4. If the adaptive forces of creation through evolution were truly at work, species would continue to form and their numbers would _____ not decrease. So why have so many disappeared?

5. Without species _____, adaptation and survival would not be possible in a changing environment.

6. The exposure to mutation-causing agents all these many years would be equivalent to millions of years of exposure in the wild, yet not one _____ of fly has been created.

Answers: repetitious, amino acids, harmony, increase, diversity, new and different species

Chapter Five

Mathematical Revelations

If the whole universe is amenable to mathematical analysis, then is there any evidence that such also relates to our own design? And if so, is there any evidence that a creator God had anything to do with it?

Did these relationships just fall into place? Or is there evidence for "divine design"? If divine design, is there any "Holy Book" that reveals a mathematical genius was involved?

Dr. Ivan Panin, a Russian mathematician and scholar of Hebrew and Greek in the early 1900s, wrote about a mathematical structure running through the Hebrew and Greek text of the Bible.

Dr. Panin was not the first to describe this mathematical structure running through the Bible. Browne in his *Ordo Saeculoreum*, Grant in his *Numbers of the Bible*, and Bullinger in his *Numbers of the Scriptures* also described numeric features found in the Bible.

Knowledge of the Hebrew letters, having a mystical significance, has been known since ancient times. The study of Jewish mysticism, relating to the numerical revelations, is known as *Gematria*. *Gematria* involves finding the hidden meanings of the numerical value of words. Generally, this numerical value points to something or to someone or some event.

More recently, it has been proposed that through "equidistant letter sequences" the Hebrew Old Testament Bible forecasts the future. This was the basis of Drosnin's 1997 bestseller *The Bible Code* (New York: Simon & Schuster). It is said that the Hebrew Bible has encoded into it messages, modern-day events, and persons revealed by these numerical relationships. Such findings, however, are subject to interpretation. Hebrew words can have many different meanings, depending on how they are used.

Equidistant letter sequencing can lead to many different interpretations, including some that are not so edifying. Like the *Gematria*, equidistant letter sequencing may require inspirational word associations to render inspirational messages. The study could itself be a trial of faith for the individual. Like life, good and bad can be derived from their study depending on the associations one seeks out.

It was not until the advent of the computer that the extent of these revelations was known. It is interesting to note that in the book of Daniel, Daniel was told that these things would not be revealed until the last days when knowledge will increase: *"But you, Daniel, close up and seal the words of the scroll until the time of the end. Many will go here and there to increase knowledge." (Daniel 12:4 NKJV)**

The computational power of computers has only now allowed us to gain insight from the numerical revelations in the Hebrew Bible. But it was Panin who discovered that the same phenomenon exist in the Greek New Testament.

Dr. Panin found that while the Hebrew text had been well-preserved. The Greek text, while still revealing an identical mathematical structure, had been edited by individuals not so interested in preserving each letter as were the Hebrew scribes and obscured this incredible relationship.

Dr. Panin is said to have used the edition of Westcott and Hort as his primary text. Some argue that these translations are not reliable. The fact is that Dr. Panin used many other alternative sources. This would make more sense. A person putting together a puzzle needs to look at all the pieces to see which one fits. Otherwise, one may never be able to put the puzzle together.

Variants (which are in the great majority spelling and other insignificant issues) have no effect on the doctrinal teachings put forth by Christ and His followers. Dr. Panin set out to rectify the numerical patterns by rewriting the text while maintaining the mathematical structure he had discovered in the Hebrew Scriptures.

Dr. Panin, while maintaining the purity of the text, put together the *Numerical Greek New Testament* (The Book Society of Canada Limited, Agincourt, Ontario, Canada, reprinted 1974). Panin found that every letter of the Hebrew and Greek manuscripts occupied a very special place in the sequence of letters of the Hebrew Old Testament and in the Greek New Testament of the Bible.[11]

The Hebrew and Greek languages have a common characteristic; they do not have numbers. Each character of their alphabet represents not only a certain enunciation but also represents a specific number.

Both languages have no separate symbol for numbers. Each letter has a numerical value. Dr. Panin through his work demonstrated that either each writer of the

Hebrew and Greek Scriptures was both a literary and mathematical genius or was guided by a force that was pervasive and omnipresent throughout the hundreds of years that the Scriptures were being written.

Dr. Panin was able to show the existence of a uniform design of complex numerical series, relationships, sequences, and combinations in the original Hebrew and Greek Scriptures. He was unable to demonstrate this same phenomenon in non-scriptural Hebrew and Greek Classics or in the Apocryphal books added at a later date by the church.

An example of Dr. Panin's findings was the discovery that the sum of the numerical characters – the letters of the sentences which start with nouns and pronouns in both the Hebrew and Greek Scriptures – add up to a number that is divisible by seven, the number that is said to be the number of God.[12]

The following table (Table 1) shows the Hebrew and Greek alphabets and their corresponding numerical and place values. The value of a word is determined by adding up the values of each letter. The order of the letters does not change its value. Generally, however, the numbers are written the largest numeral first, and with the fewest possible letters.

Since Hebrew is written and read from right to left, the largest numeral would be on the right. For example, the number fourteen (14) would be "יד" or Yod-dalet. Exceptions to this are the numbers 15 and 16 which would render the Tetragrammaton, the letters representing the name of God "יהוה", and thus are written as 9+6 "טו" tet-vav and tet-zayin "טז."

Dr. Panin showed that there were numerical patterns dealing with the numeral and place values of the Hebrew and Greek letters in both the Hebrew Old Testament and in the Greek New Testament.

When one looks at the derivations and sequences that Mr. Panin was able to come up with, one has to be impressed that he could do all of this without the aid of computers. However, the important thing of all this is not Panin's skill or whether he tweaked the numbers or not but the nature of the Bible. The Bible words and letters have numerical relationships much like most of the natural world.

There are many books being written about the various numerical relationships, their meanings, and revelations. What the words mean or how that meaning comes about is subject to interpretation, and one should not rely on interpretations taken out of context. Without the vowel signs, a Hebrew root word could have many different meanings, permitting individuals to alter the meaning to suit their purpose.

In his commentary about the works of Dr. Ivan Panin entitled *Absolute Mathematical Proofs of the Divine Inspiration of the Bible*, Dr. Keith L. Brooks wrote:

".....Many of the scripture writers were ordinary men chosen from very ordinary walks of life, having little to no schooling. If Matthew, Mark, Luke or John had attempted to write by unaided human wisdom, and produced the harmonious numeric features found throughout their books, and in each topic of their books, how long would it have taken them? Remember that with each additional sentence the difficulty of constructing on this plan increases in arithmetical and geometrical progression, for they contrive to write each paragraph so as to develop constantly fixed numeric relations to what goes before and after.

Table 1   Numerical Values Chart

Hebrew alefbet and its numerical value				Greek alphabet and its numerical value				Derivative Phoenician	
Letter	Name	Value	sound	Letter C/sc	Name	Value	sound	letter/name	value
א	alef	1	silent	A α	Alpha	1	a	Aleph	1
ב	bet	2	b or v	B β	Beta	2	b	Beth	2
ג	gimel	3	g	Γ γ	Gamma	3	g	Gimel	3
ד	dalet	4	d	Δ δ	Delta	4	d	Daleth	4
ה	he	5	h	E ε	Epsilon	5	e	He	5
ו	vav	6	v	Z ζ	Zeta	7	zd	Zayin	7
ז	zayin	7	z	H η	Eta	8	i	Heth	8
ח	het	8	he/ch	Θ θ	Theta	9	th	Teth	9
ט	tet	9	t	I ι	Iota	10	i	Yodh	10
י	yod	10	y/j	K κ	Kappa	20	k	Kaph	20
כ	kaf	20	k	Λ λ	Lambda	30	l	Lamedh	30
ך	khaf sofit		final k	M μ	Mu	40	m	Mem	40
ל	lamed	30	l	N ν	Nu	50	n	Nun	50
מ	mem	40	m	Ξ ξ	Xi	60	ks	Samekh	60
ם	mem sofit		final m	O o	Omicron	70	o	'Ayin	70
נ	nun	50	n	Π π	Pi	80	p	Pe	80
ן	nun sofit		final nun	P ρ	Rho	100	r	Resh	100
ס	samekh	60	s	Σ σ ς	Sigma	200	sound	Sin	200
ע	ayin	70	silent	T τ	Tau	300	th	Taw	300
פ	pe	80	p/f	Y υ	Upsilon	400	y	Waw	400
ף	pe sofit		final pe	Φ φ	Phi*	500	pif	*letters	500
צ	Tsade	90	ts/z	X χ	Chi*	600	kif	origin	600
ץ	Tsade sofit		final ts/z	Ψ ψ	Psi*	700	ps	questioned?	700
ק	qof	100	k	Ω ω	Omega	800	o	'Ayin	800
ר	resh	200	r						
ש	shin	300	s/sh						
ת	Tau	400	t						

"But an even more amazing feature is the number of words found in Matthew, not found in any other New Testament book, displaying elaborate numeric design. How did Matthew know that he had used words that would not be used in any of the other 26 books? He would have to have before him all these books, and would have to have written his last.

"It so happens, however, that each of the other books demonstrates the same phenomenon. Did each writer write last? If not, then was each of the writers a mind reader as well as a literary and mathematical artist, unequaled and hardly even conceivable?

"Dr. Panin proved by numerology that every book of our Hebrew and Greek Judeo-Christian Bible carries such features. And that each one is necessary to cause the numerical scheme of the entire Bible to work out correctly, and that nothing can be added or subtracted from the Hebrew and Greek Judeo-Christian Bible, as we have it, without spoiling these features.

"From the first verse of Genesis to the last verse of Revelation, the divine evidences are found. The God of nature is proved to be the God of Scripture. The quarrel of modern skeptics, therefore, is not with believers of the Bible but with God.

"The Bible begins with the Hebrew word be-re-shiyt, (בראשית) 'beginning' and ends with the Greek word *hagios*, 'holy or saint.' The Hebrew word occurs in the following books: Genesis, Exodus, Leviticus, Numbers, Deuteronomy, 2 Samuel, Isaiah, Jeremiah, Ezekiel, Hosea, Amos, Micah, Psalms, Proverbs, Job, Ecclesiastes, Daniel, Nehemiah, and 2 Chronicles. The Greek word *hagios* occurs in the following New Testament books: Matthew, Mark, Luke, John, Acts, 1st and 2nd Peter, 1st John, Jude, Romans, 1st and 2nd Corinthians, Ephesians, Philippians, Colossians, 1st and 2nd Thessalonians, Hebrews, 1st and 2nd Timothy, Titus, Philemon, and Revelation. The books are 42 in number, or six 7's.

"Take the respective number of these books in the order of their place in the Hebrew and Greek text (Table 2); their sum is 1,575 or two hundred and twenty-five 7's.

"The Judeo Christian Bible has 66 books, of which some are attributed to some author, while others are anonymous. Those which are attributed either in whole or in part to certain writers are as follows: Exodus, Leviticus, Numbers, and Deuteronomy. These are attributed at least in part to Moses, or are quoted as the works of Moses in other parts of the Bible. Isaiah, Jeremiah, Ezekiel, and the 12 Minor Prophets are attributed to the writers whose names they respectively bear. Psalms is attributed to David. Proverbs and Song of Solomon are attributed to Solomon, as is Ecclesiastes which is ascribed to "the son of David." Daniel, Ezra, and Nehemiah are attributed to their respective writers for which they are named. James, 1st and 2nd Peter, and Jude bear names of the writers. The epistles of Paul, with exception of Hebrews, are attributed to Paul. Revelation is attributed to John. The anonymous books are Genesis, Joshua, Judges, 1st and 2nd Samuel, 1st and 2nd Kings, Job, Ruth, Lamentations, Esther, 1st and 2nd Chronicles, Matthew, Mark, Luke, John, Acts, 1st, 2nd and 3rd John, and Hebrews. Of the writers named as the authors of the books of the Bible, some have ascribed to them more than one book. Moses has 4, Solomon 3, Peter 2, and Paul 13. Other writers have only one book ascribed to them.

"Now bear in mind that the books of the Bible are, in the Hebrew Received Text and the Greek Text, arranged differently from the English Bible. In the original texts, the order is as in Table 2:

Table 2		
HEBREW AND GREEK BIBLE TEXT SEQUENCE		
1. Genesis	23. Zephaniah	45. James
2. Exodus	24. Haggai	46. 1 Peter
3. Leviticus	25. Zachariah	47. 2 Peter
4. Numbers	26. Malachi	48. 1 John
5. Deuteronomy	27. Psalms	49. 2 John
6. Joshua	28. Proverbs	50. 3 John
7. Judges	29. Job	51. Jude
8. 1 Samuel	30. Song of Solomon	52. Romans
9. 2 Samuel	31. Ruth	53. 1 Corinthians
10. 1 Kings	32. Lamentations	54. 2 Corinthians
11. 2 Kings	33. Ecclesiastes	55. Galatians
12. Isaiah	34. Ester	56. Ephesians
13. Jeremiah	35. Daniel	57. Philippians
14. Ezekiel	36. Ezra	58. Collassians
15. Hosea	37. Nehemiah	59.1 Thessalonians
16. Joel	38. 1 Chronicles	60. 2 Thessalonians
17. Amos	39. 2 Chronicles	61. Hebrews
18. Obadiah	40. Matthew	62. 1 Timothy
19. Jonah	41. Mark	63. 2 Timothy
20. Micah	42. Luke	64. Titus
21. Nahum	43. John	65. Philemon
22. Habakuk	44. Acts	66. Revelation

"The number is 66, or six 11's. The anonymous books are 44, or four 11's. Of these 44, 22 or two 11's belong to writers of more than one book, and 22 or two 11's to writers of only one book. The sum of the 66 numbers is 2,211 or six 11's, which is two hundred and one 11's. This number is divided thus: the 22 books of the authors of more than one book have 946 or eighty-six 11's. The other 44 have 1,265 or one hundred and fifteen 11's.

"Of the 66 books, 21 are epistles. Their numbers are from James to Philemon, 45–65. Now the sum 2,211 for the 66 books is divided thus between epistles and non-epistles: the epistles have 1,155 or one hundred and five 11's, and the non-epistles have 1,056 or ninety-six 11's.

"Moses, David, Isaiah, Jeremiah, Hosea, Joel, and Daniel are expressly quoted in the New Testament. The number of their books is 2, 3, 4, 5, 12, 13, 15, 16, 27, and 35. The sum is 132 or twelve 11's.

"Now take the numeric values of the Bible authors (those to whom the book's title is the same as the author), by adding up the value of each letter, you get another number divisible by 11.

Table 3   Numeric Values of the Bible Authors

Moses	....	345	Zachariah	....	242
Isaiah	....	401	Malachi	....	101
Jeremiah	....	271	David	....	14
Ezekiel	....	156	Solomon	....	375
Hosea	....	381	Daniel	....	95
Joel	....	47	Ezra	....	278
Amos	....	176	Nehemiah	....	113
Obadiah	....	91	James	....	833
Jonah	....	71	Haggai	....	21
Micah	....	75	Peter	....	755
Nahum	....	104	Jude	....	685
Habakkuk	....	216	Paul	....	781
Zephaniah	....	235	John	....	1069
Total	7,931			11 X 7 X 103	

"The sum is seven hundred and twenty-one 11's. The sum of the factors 7, 11, 103 is 121, or eleven 11's. It is clearly shown that the present number of the books of the Bible is not accidental but designed. It is seen that the proportion between anonymous and non-anonymous is designed. It is seen that the number that the proportion between the number of books belongs to one writer and the number of books belonging to writers of more than one book is designed.

"These features of 7's and 11's in connection with the words and orders of the books may also be accidental, but the chance for these features of 7's and 11's happening together is one in billions. But seven is not the only number that proves of interest. There are equally interesting developments with other numbers, all of which are significant as well.

"It is seen that the proportion between epistles and non-epistles is designed. It is seen that the number of books of writers quoted in the New Testament from the Old Testament is designed. It is seen that the order of the Bible books in the Hebrew and Greek is designed. It is seen that the names of the 26 writers are designed.

"On the assumption of mere human authorship, these numeric phenomena in the order and unanimity and non-unanimity of the books are wholly unaccountable. But the assumption that a superior mathematical mind, the mathematical author of nature, has planned these numerics (unwittingly by the writers themselves), explains not only these phenomena, but also thousands of similar ones that can be brought forward."[13]

There are many attacks on the Hebrew Old Testament and the Christian New Testament, but I believe Ivan Panin demonstrated that we received what God wanted us to receive.

50

Whether we consider Numerical analysis, *Gematria*, or the Bible Code to demonstrate a mathematical connection with the universe, the strongest proof of the divine nature of the Judeo-Christian Bible, is the thousands of prophesies that it has accurately predicted (See the ending of this book for an example of some of the prophesies). The Judeo-Christian Bible is undeniably the most accurately prophetic book ever written. There are over three hundred prophecies in the Hebrew Old Testaments that were fulfilled by Jesus as evidenced by the New Testament writings.

The apocryphal books were not found to contain this numerical phenomenon, and I do not believe that the Gnostic books do either. False doctrines come from books that are not inspired by God. They are contrary to God's plan and do not contain this numerical phenomenon. These uninspired books create greater division and cause destruction of God's people. Clearly, it is the work of a destructive force, of which Paul wrote, *"All Scripture is given by inspiration of God, and is profitable for doctrine, for reproof, for correction, for instruction in righteousness, that the man of God may be complete, thoroughly equipped for every good work." (2 Timothy 3:16–17 NKJV)**

What Scripture was Paul referring to? The "Tanakh" or the Hebrew Old Testament of course! The New Testament did not even exist in Paul's time, and the Scriptures which Paul was referring to consisted of the Torah, or Law, the Neviim, or Prophets, and the Ketuvim, or The Writings. These Books at the time, and for many centuries before, were being hand recorded by Rabbinical Scribes that were required not to change one letter or make any mistake, lest they would have to start all over again.

The work was extremely tedious and took several years to complete. It is said that these scrolls were so sacred that if a fly were to land on the parchment it was considered desecrated and thus unusable and the Scribe would have to start again. Today, God's word is treated even by well-meaning men as mere paper. It is not the paper that has worth, but the message that is on it that gives it value. That is why they are considered sacred.

The teaching of doctrine, righteous conduct, and restrictions reflected in the New Testament come right out of the Hebrew Old Testament books. These were the standards and teachings that Christ Jesus lived by and are the same standards that we should live by today. To change them is to go against the will of God.

Paul warned against the perversion of God's Word, *"But even if we, or an angel from heaven, preach any other gospel to you than what we have preached to you, let him be accursed. As we have said before, so now I say again, if anyone preaches any other gospel to you than what you have received, let him be accursed. For do I now persuade men, or God? Or do I seek to please men? For if I still pleased men, I would not be a bondservant of Christ."* (Galatians 1:8–10 NKJV)*

In first Corinthians chapter 15, Paul relates a doctrine that he received from James and Peter that was well-established by the followers of Christ five years after the crucifixion of Jesus: *"For I delivered to you first of all that which I also received: that Christ died for our sins according to the Scriptures, and that He was buried, and that He rose again the third day according to the Scriptures, and that He was seen by Cephas, then by the twelve. After that He was seen by over five hundred brethren at once, of whom the greater part remain to the present, but some have fallen* *asleep. After that He was seen by James, then by all the apostles. Then last of all He was seen by me also, as by one born out of due time. For I am the least of the apostles, who am not worthy to be called an apostle, because I persecuted the church of God. But by the grace of God I am what I am, and His grace toward me was not in vain; but I labored more abundantly than they all, yet not I, but the grace of God which was with me. Therefore, whether it was I or they, so we preach and so you believed." (1 Corinthians 15:3–11 NKJV)**

This doctrine is not only strong evidence for the crucifixion death and resurrection of Jesus Christ but also contradicts the Gnostic books believed to have been written in the second and third centuries.

Chapter 5

1. Dr. Ivan Panin, a Russian mathematician and scholar of Hebrew and Greek in the early 1900s, discovered and wrote about a _____ structure running through the Hebrew and Greek text of the Bible.

2. The Hebrew and Greek languages have a common characteristic: they do not have numbers. Each character of their alphabet represents not just a certain enunciation but also _____ a specific number.

3. Dr. Panin was able to show the _____ of a uniform design of complex numerical series, relationships, sequences, and combinations in the original Hebrew and Greek scriptures.

4. These features of 7s and 11s in connection with the order and writers of the books may also be _____, but the chance for these features of 7s and 11s happening together is one in billions.

5. What Scripture was Paul referring to? The Hebrew _____ of course!

6. In first Corinthians chapter 15, Paul relates a doctrine that he received from James and Peter that was well _____ by the followers of Christ five years after the crucifixion of Jesus

Answers: mathematical, represents, existence, accidental, Old Testament, established

Chapter Six

Nature's Preoccupation with Numerical Relationships

Like the mathematical relationships found in the Bible, everything in the universe has a mathematical relationship. We can readily appreciate the effects of electricity and how some frequencies are more detrimental than other frequencies to biological forms.

Sharry Edwards, M.Ed., in her analysis of human vocal prints, has found that certain frequencies are revealing of the toxicities, biological stresses, and the overall health status of the individual. Just like no two fingerprints are alike, no two voice prints are alike. What it comes down to is that we, and all living forms, are a compilation of numerical frequencies.

A frequency is the number of vibrations, oscillations, or wave forms that occur in one second. The number of vibrations that occurs over a period of time is known as a cycle. All matter has frequency. The atomic weight of the molecules within a given substance determines its frequency. Frequency is unchanged, despite there being more of a particular molecule. What does change is the strength or the amplitude of the frequency.

An oscillation or vibration has a point or position of static equilibrium from which it moves that cancels or balances out its energy. This is the neutral point.

Energy forms, such as light energy, electromagnetic energy, and sound energy can mimic matter by vibrating at the frequency of the matter or can cancel out a frequency by vibrating at the exact opposite of the frequency, thus bringing the frequency to the point of static equilibrium.

This is the basis of energy medicine and such therapies as aroma, sound, and light therapies. Homeopathy is also based on the principal of frequency therapy as is electroacupuncture according to Voll. Instead of giving an actual substance, frequency is given in some form as a substitute for the medication. In electroacupuncture, a frequency reading can be done to identify the disease frequency causing the individuals illness. Treatment lies in bringing the frequency to equilibrium so as to reverse the disease process.

Ms. Edwards uses sound therapy based on the voice print findings to reverse the disease frequency. Ms. Edwards goes on to say: "An expression attributed to God states 'in the beginning was the word' and since sound is also frequency, God joins science in the observation that its foundation, frequency, is the basis of our universe."

Sounds in nature – whale sounds, crickets in a field, and all life forms – produce harmonious frequencies, regular and distinct patterns of sounds: a beautiful chorus, radiating from every creature on earth. We can appreciate it when we change the tempo; the wailing and the screeches become a beautiful symphony.

Quantum physics has revealed to us that frequencies form the basis for not just sound and light as we know it, but the very essence of all existence.

In the future, we should be able to analyze a person's frequencies and determine all ongoing disease processes or materials contained or carried by the individual. This may sound far-fetched, but that is exactly what we use sniffer animals for. The animals detect small traces of a given substance because of the frequency that it gives off.

Since our creator used frequency in creation, it must be the most sophisticated mode of analyzing any substance. Many are opposed to energy medicine because they lack understanding or because of financial incentives. This field, however, holds tremendous potential and merits ongoing scientific investigation.

The search for an equation that could bridge Einstein's Special Theory of Relativity and Quantum Physics has led to the String Theory which forms the basis for what all particles in the universe are composed of and how time and distance may be breached.

The String Theory is a theory of gravity, an extension of General Relativity. The String is a one-dimensional unit, oscillating lines or points that are nothing more than a frequency, in layman's term, "a word." This is exactly what John 1:1 in the Bible has been saying all along, *"In the beginning was the Word, and the Word was with God, and the Word was God." (John 1:1 NKJV)**

This is true of everything in the universe. In fact, all forms of energy are units of frequencies that drive and define all forms of matter. Like everything in nature and the universe, the Bible has a numerical pattern. Frequencies, I believe, reveal a common denominator, our Creator God.

The String Theory reveals the supernatural nature of our existence. It is a one-dimensional frequency, that is, a single numerical force or energy. This vibration determines the properties of the matter which it forms.

While purely theoretical, it reveals that we are moving closer to a concept that was previously poorly understood. Words or frequencies have power and substance. The String Theory gives greater value and understanding to what we mean when we say "the Word."

It seems Theoretical Physics is revealing many of the answers to questions about the creator God. Einstein's Theory of Relativity would lead one to determine that time is nonexistent to God. The String Theory points to the power of God's word and may well explain why distance is not an object for God.

The finding that the frequency of a particle determines the kind of particle and ultimately the kind of molecule implies that in God lies all of the frequencies that exist in the universe.

Applying the laws of entropy from physics – that everything moves from a state of greater organization to a state of lesser organization – we get the answer to the age-old question of which came first, the chicken or the egg. The chicken, being the more organized, had to have come first. Extending this to all creation, the creatures of creation had to have come into being full and complete as they are, in their most complex and organized form.

In retrospect to the point of creation, the big bang had to have been the most organized point in the universe. Imagine a point the size of a period on this page more organized than everything in the universe. This concentrated singularity contained in potential all of the information for the creation of the universe. The subsequent burst of energy dispersed in a fraction of a second producing that which we now know as the universe may in fact be the signature event of the One we know as the creator.

Chapter 6

1. Like the mathematical relationships found in the Bible, everything in the _____ has a mathematical relationship.

2. The search for an equation that could bridge Einstein's Special Theory of Relativity and Quantum Physics has led to the _____ Theory, which forms the basis for what all particles in the universe are composed of.

3. The String is a one-dimensional unit, oscillating lines or points that are nothing more than a frequency, in layman's term "a _____."

4. This is true of everything in the universe, light, sound; in fact, all forms of energy are units of _____ that drive and define all forms of matter.

5. Theoretical Physics it seems is _____ many of the answers to questions about the creator God.

6. In retrospect to the point of creation, the big bang had to have been the most _____ point in the universe

Answers: universe, String, word, frequencies, revealing, organized

Chapter Seven

The Point

You may ask: what does this have to do with the concept of an ideal body? Why review and explore these far-reaching ideas? The answer is simple. I believe the Bible reveals the only truly ideal body that ever walked on the face of the Almighty's creation.

"Who had it?" you ask. I believe the only person to have ever lived that had an ideal body was Jesus after His resurrection. Jesus, who is also called the Christ, the anointed one, or the Messiah, is the only human being recorded in reliable history to have died and to have risen from the dead in a transformed body, an ideal body.

The Gospel of John goes on to equate this Jesus with frequency, as He is also called The Word. *"In the beginning was the Word, and the Word was with God and the Word was God. He was in the beginning with God. All things were made through Him, and without Him nothing was made that was made. In Him was life and the life was the light of men. And the light shines in the darkness, and the darkness did not comprehend it." (John 1:2–4 NKJV)**

There is sufficient historical evidence that Jesus in fact came back to life after having died by crucifixion. Some have theorized that He had not really died; He had been drugged so as to appear to be dead. However, the fact remains that if anyone knew how to put someone to death, the Romans could be said to have been professionals at it.

They broke the legs of those whom they suspected of not having died. In the record of the crucifixion, they speared Jesus in the heart.

Crucifixion causes death by suffocation. The soldiers closely watch for the breathing to stop in their victims. It is not a difficult observation. I suspect that as Christ exhibited agonal breathing some soldier stabbed Him in the chest with his spear to quicken His death. Regardless, it is well - recorded that He died and on the third day, by Jewish observance, arose from the dead. It is also recorded that He appeared in a transformed body to over five thousand people, demonstrating supernatural abilities.

In the story of the Shroud of Turin, the linen suppo- sedly used to wrap the body of Christ during His burial, there is a negative image outlining the body. The image appears to have been caused by some sort of radiation emitted from the body during its revitalization. This suggests a supernatural event took place in Christ body during His transformation.

Sufficient plant spores of various plant life found only in that part of the world were found on the Shroud to place it in that location at about the time of Christ. As stated, there is evidence to suggest that an energetic transformation occurred during Christ's resurrection. The transformation gave Him supernatural abilities far beyond the abilities He had as a man. These abilities I believe would be those of an ideal body.

Some suggest that the Shroud is not authentic. The person whose image is presented has long hair. The disciple of Jesus, Paul, spoke against men having long hair. However, long hair was common in the Nazarene sect of the Jews. Jesus was called a Nazarene.

Not cutting the hair was a sign of living under a vow. In fact, the completion of the vow was often followed with the shaving of the head. Christ's vow to perform the task Father God sent Him to do was not over until after His crucifixion and resurrection.

There are also arguments concerning Paul's admonition of the covering of the head. Paul was speaking of a veil covering over the face and not specifically about the covering of the head as many would think. A veil over a man's face was disgraceful, but a woman's hair was given for such purpose. To discredit the Shroud on the grounds that the man represented had long hair fails to take into account the religious customs of the time.

What were the qualities of His resurrected body? In the few recordings of His appearance, it is apparent that Jesus had supernatural abilities beyond those that He had exhibited prior to His crucifixion.

On the road to Emmaus, Jesus demonstrated the ability to control recognition. He also was able to dematerialize and thus apparently to vanish unseen. *"Now that same day two of them were going to a village called Emmaus, about seven miles from Jerusalem. They were talking with each other about everything that had happened. As they talked and discussed these things with each other, Jesus Himself came up and walked along with them; but they were kept from recognizing Him. He asked them, 'What are you discussing together as you walk along?' They stood still, their faces downcast. One of them, named Cleopas, asked Him, 'Are you only a visitor to Jerusalem and do not know the things that have happened there in these days?' 'What things?' He asked. 'About Jesus of Nazareth,' they replied. 'He was a prophet, powerful in word and deed before God and all the people. The chief* priests and our rulers handed Him over to be sentenced to death, and they crucified Him; but we had hoped that He was the one who was going to redeem Israel. And what is more, it is the third day since all this took place. In addition, some of our women amazed us. They went to the tomb early this morning but didn't find His body. They came and told us that they had seen a vision of angels, who said He was alive. Then some of our companions went to the tomb and found it just as the women had said, but Him they did not see.' He said to them, 'How foolish you are, and how slow of heart to believe all that the prophets have spoken! Did not the Christ have to suffer these things and then enter His glory?' And beginning with Moses and all the Prophets, He explained to them what was said in all the Scriptures concerning Himself. As they approached the village to which they were going, Jesus acted as if He were going farther. But they urged Him strongly, 'Stay with us, for it is nearly evening; the day is almost over.' So He went in to stay with them. When He was at the table with them, He took bread, gave thanks, broke it, and began to give it to them. Then their eyes were opened and they recognized Him, and He disappeared from their sight. They asked each other, 'Were not our hearts burning within us while He talked with us on the road and opened the Scriptures to us?'" (Luke 24:13–32 NKJV)*

In a gathering of the disciples, Jesus demonstrated the ability to materialize even through solid walls. He showed the disciples the wounds in His hands and His feet and the stab wound in His chest. Jesus demonstrated that He was not a spirit but was flesh and ate fish and honeycomb in their presence to prove it.

In departing from the disciples, Jesus levitated Himself from their presence into the heavens. "While they were still talking about this, Jesus Himself stood among them and said to them, 'Peace be with you.' They were startled and *frightened, thinking they saw a ghost. He said to them, 'Why are you troubled, and why do doubts rise in your minds? Look at My hands and My feet. It is I Myself! Touch Me and see; a ghost does not have flesh and bones, as you see I have.' When He had said this, He showed them His hands and feet. And while they still did not believe it because of joy and amazement, He asked them, 'Do you have anything here to eat?' They gave Him a piece of broiled fish, and He took it and ate it in their presence. He said to them, 'This is what I told you while I was still with you: Everything must be fulfilled that is written about Me in the Law of Moses, the Prophets and the Psalms.' Then He opened their minds so they could understand the Scriptures. He told them, 'This is what is written: The Christ will suffer and rise from the dead on the third day, and repentance and forgiveness of sins will be preached in His name to all nations, beginning at Jerusalem. You are witnesses of these things. I am going to send you what My Father has promised; but stay in the city until you have been clothed with power from on high.' When He had led them out to the vicinity of Bethany, He lifted up His hands and blessed them. While He was blessing them, He left them and was taken up into heaven. Then they worshiped Him and returned to Jerusalem with great joy. And they stayed continually at the temple, praising God."* (Luke 24:36–51 NKJV)*

Jesus demonstrated that He was not bound by natural laws and possessed supernatural abilities. His greatest feat was that of defeating death. The resurrection of Jesus was the one feat that demonstrated the superiority of Jesus over all prophets and religious leaders before Him or since.

The transformation of Jesus that occurred with His resurrection resulted in a body capable of ingesting food and not restricted by material barriers, a body that in accordance with His teachings would never die but would continue to live for all eternity.

The question is why – if Jesus was sent by God the Father – why was He sent, what was His mission, and why did He preach that anyone that believed in Him would join Him and be like Him even if they died?

Saul, a nonbeliever, encountered the resurrected Jesus while en route to persecute the disciples. Jesus revealed Himself to Saul as a blinding light, an energetic force.

Saul became a believer and was renamed Paul. As a result of this experience, Saul converted, and as Paul, he wrote many of the books found in the New Testament.

Like many of the Apostles, Paul was enlightened by the Spirit of Jesus. In his letter to the Corinthians, Paul wrote, *"Now when all things are made subject to Him (Jesus), then the Son Himself will also be subject to Him who put all things under Him, that God may be all in all."* (1 Corinthians 15:28 NKJV)*

*"For it pleased the Father that in Him all the fullness should dwell, and by Him to reconcile all things to Himself, by Him, whether things on earth or things in heaven, having made peace through the blood of His cross." (Colossians 1:19–20 NKJV)** God used Jesus to reconcile all things to Himself, that is, to make all things good, to recoup His glory.

Jesus' mission was to restore all things back to the Father, to bring all things under subjugation for Father God. In the end, Jesus will put all things including Himself under the Father.

Many teach that Jesus came to save us. But our salvation is a secondary benefit of our joining Jesus in His mission to restore the Glory to the Father.

Jesus came for a purpose, but His purpose was not as many would claim. What He does in the end reveals His purpose and His mission: to restore the Glory to the Father. The Scriptures tell us that we are His reward for a job well done. *"God, who at various times and in various ways spoke in times past to the fathers by the prophets, has in these last days spoken to us by His Son, whom He has appointed heir of all things, through whom also He made the worlds; who being the brightness of His glory and the express image of His person, and upholding all things by His power, when He had Himself purged our sins, sat down at the right hand of the Majesty on high, having become so much better than the angels, as He has by inheritance obtained a more excellent name than they." (Hebrews 1:1–4 NKJV)**

Chapter 7

1. Jesus, who is also called the Christ, the anointed one, or the Messiah, is the only human being recorded in reliable history to have _____ and to have risen from the dead in a transformed body, an ideal body.

2. Regardless, it is well-recorded that He died and on the third day, by Jewish observance, arose from the dead, and appeared in a transformed body to over five _____ people, demonstrating supernatural abilities.

3. In the few recordings of His appearance, it is apparent that Jesus had _____ abilities beyond those that He had exhibited prior to His crucifixion.

4. In a gathering of the disciples, Jesus demonstrated the ability to _____ even through solid walls.

5. Jesus demonstrated that He was not a _____ but was flesh and ate fish and honeycomb in their presence to prove it.

6. Jesus' mission was to _____ all things back to the Father, to bring all things under subjugation for Father God.

Answers: died, thousand, supernatural, materialize, spirit, restore

Chapter Eight

The Glory Recaptured

The Bible tells us that God's kingdom is occupied by a host of heavenly bodies, angels, and archangels who worship God their creator. One chief angel identified by the prophet Isaiah as Lucifer, *"....O Lucifer son of the morning!..." (Isaiah 14:12 NKJV)** Lucifer, meaning angel of light or brightness of morning, rebelled against God. *"How you are fallen from heaven, O Lucifer, son of the morning! How you are cut down to the ground, you who weakened the nations! For you have said in your heart: I will ascend into heaven, I will exalt my throne above the stars of God; I will also sit in the mount of the congregation, on the farthest side of the north; I will ascend above the heights of the clouds, I will be like the Most High." (Isaiah 14:12–14 NKJV)**

Lucifer, wanting to be as God, was thrown out of Heaven. Leaving with his followers consisting of one-third of God's angels, they took up habitation on the earth wandering about as spiritual disembodied beings, always aspiring to overthrow God and any plan God may have.

Ezekiel, the prophet, prophesied concerning this rebel Lucifer and one of the many men whose body he would possess. He was not referring to a man but to Lucifer who ruled through a man, the prince of Tyre. *"...The word of the Lord came to me again saying, 'Son of man, say to the prince of Tyre; thus says the Lord God: "Because your heart is lifted up," and you say, 'I am a god, I sit in the seat of gods, In the midst of the seas, Yet you are a man, and not a* *god, Though you set your heart as the heart of god. Behold you are wiser than Daniel; there is no secret that that can be hidden from you! With your wisdom and your understanding you have gained riches for yourself, and gathered gold and silver into your treasures; By your great wisdom in trade you have increased your riches, and your heart is lifted up because of your riches,' Therefore thus says the Lord God: 'Because you have set your heart as the heart of god, Behold I will bring strangers against you, The most terrible of the nations; and they shall draw their swords against the beauty of your wisdom, and defile your splendor. They shall throw you down into the Pit, and you shall die the death of the slain in the midst of the seas.' 'Will you still say before him who slays you, I am a god? But you shall be a man, and not a god, in the hand of him who slays you, you shall die the death of the uncircumcised by the hand of the aliens; For I have spoken,' says the Lord God." (Ezekiel 28:1–10 NKJV)**

God was speaking to a man possessed by Lucifer. Lucifer, while a great angel, was still a creation of God. His name implies angel of light. He may have been called such because he possessed great knowledge, as light frequently is said to represent being enlightened or possessing knowledge. Ezekiel credits him with being wiser than Daniel. This knowledge made him seem as a god to his subordinate angels.

Lucifer, feeling that he had the knowledge of God, was puffed up with pride. Wanting to be as God, he rebelled in an attempt to displace his creator. This rebellion was a disgraceful act against God, an attempt to steal God's glory. God would have to recoup this glory in such a fashion that would demonstrate that even the great knowledge of Lucifer is foolishness in comparison to God's knowledge and understanding.

But if God is all-knowing and sees all the future and the past, how could this be? How could an all-knowing God permit someone to disgrace Him? Or had He another plan and a different purpose which this rebellion was in fact a part of?

The word God implies an entity that is deserving of worship. But worship obtained by force is not worship at all. It must come voluntarily from the source to be true worship, especially if one is speaking of a loving God. If God were to have to force His angels to be obedient, He would not be God but a tyrant, which would put to question whether He deserves worship at all.

His majesty is in the sincere worship of His subjects who love Him for who He is, their creator, and not because He could destroy or vanish them. God permitted one that would rebel knowing that this would draw a line between His loyal subjects, the true worshippers, and the deceitful followers.

This is a "mystery, which from the beginning of the ages has been hidden in God who created all things..." which was revealed to Paul: *"...and to make all see what is the fellowship of the mystery, which from the beginning of the ages has been hidden in God who created all things through Jesus Christ." (Ephesians 3:9 NKJV)**

The free-will worship of His subjects, both heavenly and terrestrial, is of the utmost importance to our creator God. By definition, the word "God" implies a being that is freely and willingly worshiped by His servants, His creation. Without it, God would not be God. Thus it is demonstrated that God knew from the "beginning" that such a rebellion would happen and prepared a plan, which Paul claimed was the "mystery" revealed to him.

What was God's plan to gain the loyalty of His subjects? He would show His subjects His manifold wisdom in such a way that they would marvel and know that He is worthy of their worship.

With Lucifer rebelling, God chose lowly man to show Lucifer up. In the letter to the Ephesians chapter 3, verse 10, Paul wrote: *"to the intent that now the manifold wisdom of God might be made known by the church (the body of believers) to the principalities and powers in the heavenly places." (Ephesians 3:10 NKJV)*

The church or the body of believers would teach God's angels a lesson of the manifold wisdom of God. How could that be? We are but lowly creatures, unworthy of even brushing the dust off the feet of the lowliest angel. But Paul states that God revealed to him that that is exactly what He was doing. He was using us to draw the line, to reveal just how much more wisdom there is in Him than that thought to be had by His challenger Lucifer.

But how would God make lowly man to show Lucifer up? How would He make man want to worship Him and disgrace Lucifer, who had been given everything and who should have been grateful for the position God had placed him in? He would do it with His love!

God has a Son. While many are ignorant about or refuse to accept it, the book of Proverbs, written by King Solomon, recognized for his wisdom some 900 years before the birth of Jesus, in chapter 30 verse 4, states: *"Who has ascended into heaven? Or who has descended from heaven? Who has gathered the wind in His fist? Who has bound the waters in a garment? Who has established the ends of the earth? What is His name, and what is His Son's name, if you know?" (Proverbs 30:4 NKJV)*

Isaiah describes the right hand of God, presumed to be speaking of this same "Son of God" of Proverbs 30:4, in Isaiah 48 verse 13: *"Indeed My hand has laid the foundation of the earth and My right hand has stretched out the heavens; when I call out to them, they stand up together."* (Isaiah 48:13 NKJV)* The other hand spoken of in this verse is considered to be the Holy Spirit.

God sent a part of Himself to demonstrate His love to us that whoever finds Him finds life as demonstrated in Proverbs chapter 8 verses 22 to 36. *"The Lord possessed me at the beginning of His way, Before His works of old. I have been established from everlasting. From the beginning, before there was ever an earth. When there were no depths I was brought forth. When there were no fountains abounding with water, before the mountains were settled, before the hills, I was brought forth; while as yet He had not made the earth or the fields, or the primal dust of the world. When He prepared the heavens, I was there, When He drew a circle on the face of the deep, When He established the clouds above, When He strengthened the fountains of the deep, When He assigned to the sea its limit, So that the waters would not transgress His command, When He marked out the foundations of the earth, Then I was beside Him as a master craftsman; And I was daily His delight, Rejoicing always before Him, Rejoicing in His inhabited world, And my delight was with the sons of men. Now therefore, listen to me, my children, for blessed are those who keep my ways. Hear instruction and be wise, and do not disdain it. Blessed is the man who listens to me, Watching daily at my gates, Waiting at the posts of my doors. For whoever finds me finds life, and obtains favor from the Lord; But he who sins against me wrongs his own soul; All those who hate me love death."* (Proverbs 8:22–36 NKJV)*

God brought forth a part of Himself. The implication is that this craftsman was present from the beginning with God. This craftsman, it goes on, was brought forth to bring revelation and a way of obtaining favor from God. *"Whoever finds me finds life"* means more than just to be among the living. It implies living forever. For by definition, this "life" could not mean anything less than the life that this craftsman would Himself have.

Who is this craftsman? This craftsman is Jesus. It was Jesus who claimed, *"Before Abraham was I AM." (John 8:58 NKJV)** The disciples of Jesus frequently credited Jesus with the creation. *"All things were made through Him, and by Him, and without Him nothing was made that was made." (John 1:3 NKJV)** Also, as previously demonstrated in Paul's letter in Ephesians 3:9, Paul claimed all things were created through Jesus.

Jesus came on a mission. His mission was to recoup the glory of God taken by Lucifer or — as he later became known as — "Satan." Satan is the name given to him after rebelling. Satan means deceiver, the great deceiver.

The objective of the mission of Jesus can readily be identified when one understands what Jesus does in the end upon completing His mission. In the end, Jesus gives everything to the Father, as Paul states in 1st Corinthians: *"Now when all things are made subject to Him, then the Son Himself will also be subject to Him who put all things under Him that God may be all in all." (1 Corinthians 15:28 NKJV)**

Many religious leaders claim that Jesus came to save us, to give us eternal life. While the net effect is our salvation, as defined by us acquiring eternal life, the acquiring of eternal life is a gift that we receive for joining Jesus in His mission.

Imagine the angels of God watching down in amazement, wondering: He (God) is going to do what with whom? How could that be? No doubt that is why Jesus said: *"I say to you likewise there will be more joy in heaven over one sinner who repents than over ninety-nine just persons who need no repentance." (Luke 15:7 NKJV)**

Our decision to accept Jesus brings peace to us and is a blow to Satan. It also serves as a lesson to the heavenly beings. That is why it states, *"For it pleased the Father that in Him all the fullness should dwell, and by Him to reconcile all things to Himself, by Him, whether things on earth or things in heaven, having made peace through the blood of His cross." (Colossians 1:19–20 NKJV)**

Each person that repents shows up Lucifer's rebellion, a significant blow since it comes from such insignificant beings, beings that should not know better, showing up the one who considers that he knows it all. No wonder there is such rejoicing in heaven.

Chapter 8

1. Lucifer wanting to be as God was thrown out of Heaven. Leaving with his followers consisting of one-third of God's angels, they took up _____ on the earth, wandering about as spiritual disembodied beings.

2. But if God is all knowing and sees all the future and the past, how could this be, how could an all-knowing God permit someone to _____ Him or had He another plan and a different purpose which this rebellion fell into?

3. With Lucifer rebelling, God chose lowly _____ to show Lucifer up.

4. God sent a part of _____ to demonstrate His love to us that whoever finds Him finds life as demonstrated in Proverbs chapter 8.

5. For by definition this "life" could not mean anything less than the life that this _____ would have.

6. Imagine the _____ of God watching down in amazement, wondering: He (God) is going to do what with whom? How could that be?

Answers: habitation, disgrace, man, Himself, craftsman, angels

Chapter Nine

The Perfect Jesus

Jesus was perfect under the law of God, but His earthly body was far from ideal. He hungered. He thirsted. He fatigued. He had to rest. He was limited as we today are limited. But by God's standard He was perfect. Jesus had to be perfect to fit into God's Kingdom plans.

Jesus was perfect in obedience. He had to be. A perfect God could only receive a perfect sacrifice. No other person deified by man who ever lived could claim to be perfect. But Jesus is recorded in the Bible as being perfect. He had to be. If He were to be sacrificed to God as the sacrificial lamb, He would have to be perfect.

It would be unacceptable to come for the purpose of restoring God's glory and to dishonor Him with a less than perfect sacrifice. That is why He had to be perfect. Jesus Himself said, "Be perfect as my Father in heaven is perfect," in effect pronouncing Himself as perfect.

God as supreme Judge must punish sin, more so than a worldly judge must punish crime. Jesus voluntarily gave Himself to be punished for our sins that we through His sacrifice may receive justification and forgiveness of sin to fulfill God's plan. To do this, Jesus had to be perfect.

Richard Booker, in his book *Jesus in the Feast of Israel*, superbly demonstrates the prophetic messages in the

Israeli feast and how they relate to the coming of the Messiah.

For 1,500 years prior to the earthly birth of Jesus, the Jews had been celebrating the Feast of Passover by killing a lamb and offering it as a sacrifice to God. They would do this every year, knowing that their sins would be covered for one more year.

The blood of an animal could only cover their sins. It could not take their sins away. In view of this, there arose prophets sent by God to explain to the people that, one day in the future, a human lamb would come who would deal with the problem of sin and death once and for all.

The prophet Isaiah spoke of the suffering this human lamb would experience some 700 years before Jesus' birth. Isaiah wrote a very clear and vivid description, which is recorded for us in Isaiah, chapter 53: *"Who has believed our report? And to whom has the arm of the Lord been revealed? For He shall grow up before Him as a tender plant, And as a root out of dry ground; He has no form or comeliness; And when we see Him, There is no beauty that we should desire of Him. He is despised and rejected by men, a man of sorrows and acquainted with grief. And we hid, as if it were our faces from Him; He was despised and we did not esteem Him. Surely He has borne our grief and carried our sorrows. Yet we esteem Him stricken, smitten by God, and afflicted. But He was wounded for our transgressions, He was bruised for our iniquities; the chastisement for our peace was upon Him, and by His stripes we are healed. All we like sheep have gone astray; we have turned, every one, to his own way; And the Lord has laid on Him the iniquity of us all. He was oppressed and He was afflicted, Yet He opened not His mouth; He was led as a lamb to slaughter, And as a sheep before its shearers is silent, So He opened* not His Mouth. He was taken from prison and from judgment, And who will declare His generation? For He was cut off from the land of the living; For the transgressions of My people He was stricken. And they made His grave with the wicked, But with the rich at His death, Because He had done no violence, nor was any deceit in His mouth. Yet it pleased the Lord to bruise Him; He has put Him to grief. When You make His soul an offering for sin He shall see His seed, He shall prolong His days, And the pleasure of the Lord shall prosper in His hand. He shall see the labor of His soul and be satisfied. By His knowledge My righteous Servant shall justify many. For He shall bear their iniquities, therefore I will divide Him a portion with the great, And He shall divide the spoil with the strong. Because He poured out His soul unto death, And He was numbered with the transgressors; And He bore the sin of many, And made intercession for the transgressors." (Isaiah 53 NKJV)*

As the time came for this human lamb to be sacrificed, God sent one last prophet to help the people to recognize Him. This prophet was John the Baptist, a cousin and contemporary of Jesus. John introduced Jesus with these words, "Behold! The Lamb of God who takes away the sin of the world." (John 1:29 NKJV)*

John identified Jesus as the human lamb Isaiah spoke of who would give His life for the sins of the world. For this purpose, Jesus was born; "And she will bring forth a Son, and you shall call His name Jesus, for He will save His people from their sins." (Matthew 1:21 NKJV)*

Because of their religious sacrifices, the Jews understood the significance of John's statements concerning Jesus. Jesus fulfilled the Feast of Passover in His crucifixion. This was the reason for His human birth.

The entire life of Jesus was predestined so that He would fulfill this purpose exactly as God had instructed the Jews to practice for 1,500 years prior to Jesus.

In view of this, as the time approached for Him to be crucified, Jesus arranged His activities around the events associated with the selection, testing, and death of the Passover lamb. In this way, the Jewish people would understand who He was and what He was doing.

Jesus was set aside to be sacrificed — examined and crucified — on the exact month, day, and hour that the Jews had been handling the lambs for 1,500 years in keeping with the Feast of Passover.

God established the Passover feast in Egypt on the tenth day of the month of Nisan. He instructed the Jews to set aside their lambs on the tenth day of the month of Nisan. In the New Testament, we learn that it was the tenth day of the month of Nisan when Jesus entered Jerusalem.

In John 12:1, we find that Jesus came to the town of Bethany six days before the Passover. John writes, *"Then six days before Passover, Jesus came to Bethany." (John 12:1 NKJV)**

Since Passover was celebrated on the fourteenth, this would mean that Jesus came to Bethany on the ninth. John then gives us further information to show us that the ninth was on a Saturday. He goes on to say, *"The next day a multitude that had come to the feast, when they heard that Jesus was coming to Jerusalem, took branches of palm trees and went out to meet Him, and cried out: 'Hosanna! Blessed is He who comes in the name of the Lord! The King of Israel!'" (John 12:12–13 NKJV)** John states that it was the next day when Jesus rode into Jerusalem and was greeted by the cheering crowds. This, of course, is what the Christian church has historically referred to as Palm Sunday.

Jesus was in Bethany on Saturday, the ninth of Nisan. The next day was Sunday, the tenth of Nisan. Jesus entered Jerusalem to be set aside as the human Lamb of God on the exact date that God told the Jews to set aside their lambs back in Egypt.

The purpose for setting aside the Lamb was so that they could be observed to make sure that they were without defect or disease or, as some say, without spot or blemish. This lamb was to be offered up to God. God is perfect. The lamb also would have to be perfect. An imperfect animal would be unacceptable. So the Jews observed and inspected the lamb for five days to make sure that it was faultless.

Likewise, Jesus, the human lamb, was evaluated for five days by the religious leaders. They questioned His authority. They interrogated Him with trick questions, hoping He would somehow give a wrong answer that they would be able to use against Him. However, Jesus responded to them perfectly. They could not find anything wrong with Him. *"Now when He came into the temple, the chief priests and the elders of the people confronted Him as He was teaching, and said, 'By what authority are You doing these things? And who gave You this authority?' But Jesus answered and said to them, 'I also will ask you one thing, which if you tell Me, I likewise will tell you by what authority I do these things: The baptism of John, where was it from? From heaven or from men?' And they reasoned among themselves, saying, 'If we say, "From heaven," He will say to us, "Why then did you not believe him?" But if we say, "From men," we fear the multitude, for all count John as a prophet.' So they answered Jesus and said, 'We do not* know.' And He said to them, 'Neither will I tell you by what authority I do these things.' (Matthew 21:23–27 NKJV)* The same day the Sadducees, who say there is no resurrection, came to Him and asked Him, saying: 'Teacher, Moses said that if a man dies, having no children, his brother shall marry his wife and raise up offspring for his brother. Now there were with us seven brothers. The first died after he had married, and having no offspring, left his wife to his brother. Likewise the second also, and the third, even to the seventh. Last of all the woman died also. Therefore, in the resurrection, whose wife of the seven will she be? For they all had her.' Jesus answered and said to them, 'You are mistaken, not knowing the Scriptures nor the power of God. For in the resurrection they neither marry nor are given in marriage, but are like angels of God in heaven. But concerning the resurrection of the dead, have you not read what was spoken to you by God, saying, "I am the God of Abraham, the God of Isaac, and the God of Jacob?" God is not the God of the dead, but of the living.' And when the multitudes heard this, they were astonished at His teaching. But when the Pharisees heard that He had silenced the Sadducees, they gathered together. Then one of them, a lawyer, asked Him a question, testing Him, and saying, 'Teacher, which is the great commandment in the law?' Jesus said to him, "You shall love the LORD your God with all your heart, with all your soul, and with all your mind." This is the first and great commandment. And the second is like it: "You shall love your neighbor as yourself." On these two commandments hang all the Law and the Prophets.' While the Pharisees were gathered together, Jesus asked them, saying, 'What do you think about the Christ? Whose Son is He?' They said to Him, 'The Son of David.' He said to them, 'How then does David in the Spirit call Him "Lord," saying: "The LORD said to my Lord, 'Sit at My right hand, Till I make Your enemies Your footstool?'" If David then calls Him

"Lord," how is He his Son?" And no one was able to answer Him a word, nor from that day on did anyone dare question Him anymore. (Matthew 22:23–45 NKJV)* Finally in desperation they took Jesus to the Roman governor, whose name was Pilate, hoping he could find something wrong with Him. But after interrogating and beating Jesus, Pilate then went out again, and said to them, 'Behold, I am bringing Him out to you, that you may know that I find no fault in Him.'" (John 19:4 NKJV)*

This all happened in the five-day period from the tenth to the fourteenth while the Jews were observing their lambs for the sacrificial offering.

Jesus was crucified on the fourteenth day of Nisan, on the very same day and at the very same time of day as the sacrificial lambs were being sacrificed. At the same hour, the Jews were preparing their lambs for sacrifice, Jesus was nailed to the cross. Mark wrote: "Now it was the third hour, and they crucified Him." (Mark 15:25 NKJV)* The third hour is nine o'clock in the morning, the time the lambs were being readied for their sacrifice.

Then at three o'clock, as the people were praising God and slaughtering the lambs, Jesus died. Mark was careful to note the time and wrote that it was the ninth hour (three o'clock Jewish time), when Jesus breathed His last breath.[14] "Now when the sixth hour had come, there was darkness over the whole land until the ninth hour. And at the ninth hour Jesus cried out with a loud voice, saying, 'Eloi, Eloi, lama sabachthani?' which is translated, 'My God, My God, why have You forsaken Me?' Some of those who stood by, when they heard that, said, 'Look, He is calling for Elijah!' Then someone ran and filled a sponge full of sour wine, put it on a reed, and offered it to Him to drink, saying, 'Let Him alone; let us see if Elijah will come to take Him down.' And Jesus cried out with a loud voice, and breathed His last." (Mark 15:33–37 NKJV)*

Anyone who reads about the life of Jesus in the Bible can only conclude that His life was consistently the purest of anyone in recorded history. None of His challengers were able to bring any valid charges against Him with respect to the laws of God.

Contrary to all of the great religious leaders in history – leaders such as Buddha, Krishna, Mohammed, and the great prophets – all of them struggled with staying free of the perceived wrongs of their day at some point or another in their lives.

The Koran documents Moses asking for forgiveness after slaying the Egyptian (Surah 28, 16) and Abraham asking for forgiveness on the Day of Judgment (Surah 26, 82). Mohammed was told to ask for forgiveness for his faults in Surah 47 and 48.

Krishna is recorded in the Bhagavad-Gita as having encounters with the milkmaids, and Buddha's multiple incarnations imply having lived imperfect lives.[15] Jesus, however, was recognized by the people of His time as being faultless. Jesus was perfect before God, unlike any man deified by man.

Jesus did not come seeking the truth. He claimed He was the truth. This one claim puts Him above all others. Jesus said: "I am the way, the truth, and the life. No one comes to the Father except through Me." (John 14:6 NKJV)* In fact, He said He was more than just the way. He said, "I and My Father are one." (John 10:30 NKJV)*

Regardless of how you interpret this, Jesus could not have said these things unless they had some profound significance. This places Him in a category far above any prophet or religious leader in history.

Jesus could still the wind, heal the sick, make fine wine from water, multiply bread loaves, raise the dead, and walk on water. He was either who He said He was, or He was the greatest imposter to have ever walked the Earth. Yet, He claimed He came to die for our sins. When the governor of Judea, Pontius Pilate, told Him: *"Do You not know that I have authority to release You, and I have authority to crucify You?"* Jesus answered, *"You would have no authority over Me, unless it had been given from above."* (John 19:10–11 NKJV)*

When Jesus was arrested and one of His disciples tried to defend Him drawing his sword and striking the servant of the high priest, cutting off his ear, Jesus stopped him, saying: *"Put your sword in its place, for all who take the sword will perish by the sword. Or do you not think that I cannot now pray to my Father, and He will provide Me with more than twelve legions of angels? How then could the Scriptures be fulfilled, that it must happen thus?"* (Matthew 26:52–54 NKJV)*

The Gospel accounts of the arrest, trials, and crucifixion of Jesus indicate that He made no attempt to defend Himself or to escape His situation. Like it is written in Isaiah: *"He was oppressed and He was afflicted, Yet He opened not His mouth; He was led as a lamb to the slaughter, And as a sheep before its shearers is silent, So He opened not His mouth."* (Isaiah 53:7 NKJV)*

Jesus came to die as God's sacrificial Lamb for our sins. In dying, He demonstrated God's love for us and

God's desire for us to love Him. In John 3:16 it states: *"For God so loved the world that He gave His only begotten Son that whoever believes in Him shall not perish but have eternal life." (John 3:16 NKJV)** This passage indicates that Jesus is begotten, that is, He is a part of the Father, and that the Father loves us enough to give us a part of Himself, His Son, and that for our acceptance of this gift, He rewards us with eternal life.

This may sound simplistic, but when one looks at the story of Abraham, one can understand God's desire for us to love Him as much as He loves us. God told Abraham to sacrifice his son to Him: *"Then He said, Take now your son, your only son Isaac, whom you love, and go to the land of Moriah, and offer him there as a burnt offering on one of the mountains of which I shall tell you." (Genesis 22:2 NKJV)** God was asking of Abraham what He Himself was willing to give to mankind, His son.

Abraham understood this and knew that he was to demonstrate to God that he loved Him in like manner. Jesus on commenting on Abraham said: *"Your father Abraham rejoiced to see My day, and he saw it and was glad." (John 8:56 NKJV)**

Abraham was obedient to God as it states: *"And Abraham stretched out his hand and took the knife to slay his son. But the angel of the Lord called to him from heaven and said, 'Abraham, Abraham!' So he said, 'Here I am.' And He said, 'Do not lay your hand on the lad, or do anything to him; for now I know that you fear God, since you have not withheld your son, your only son, from Me.'" (Genesis 22:10–12 NKJV)**

Abraham was obedient and feared God. But what does it mean when it says, "he feared God"? Was

Abraham afraid of God, fearful of what disaster God could have poured down on him? God gave him his son. Now, He wanted Abraham to give his son back.

What was it that God really wanted? God desired to be the priority in Abraham's life! He wanted His relationship with Abraham to be the most precious thing in Abraham's possession, something Lucifer failed to give God! This is the same thing God would have with each and every one of us.

In Proverbs, it states: *"The fear of the Lord is to hate evil..." (Proverbs 8:13 NKJV)** – to hate what God hates – But what does this mean? We are to abhor anything and everything that offends God. We need to appreciate who He is and what He is capable of doing and respect Him for it. Fear taken to its highest level instills intense respect. We must revere Him. That is how we should be about God.

God wants us to love Him and respect Him so much that we would not want anything to offend Him or put anything ahead of Him, not even ourselves! Abraham was the first to show Lucifer up, willing to give God his most precious possession, his son.

For being willing to give God his most prized possession, God rewarded Abraham, and not just him but all of his descendants. *"...By Myself I have sworn, says the Lord, because you have done this thing, and have not withheld your son, your only son, blessing I will bless you, and multiplying I will multiply your descendants as the stars of the heaven and as the sand which is on the seashore; and your descendants shall possess the gate of their enemies, In your seed all nations of the earth shall be blessed, because you have obeyed My voice." (Genesis 22:16–18 NKJV)**

Even before this, while Abraham was still called Abram, God promised to keep covenant with him and to make him the father of many nations. *"As for Me, behold My covenant is with you, and you shall be a father of many nations." (Genesis 17:4 NKJV)**

Today, there are approximately fifteen million people worldwide who identify themselves as being a Jew by birth. Yet, Abraham was promised that his descendants would number *"as the stars in the heaven and as the sand, which is on the seashore..." (Genesis 22:17 NKJV)**

Where are the other people and nations of God's promise? Certainly, if God is to show Lucifer up, He would have to do it with more than one small nation. The fifteen million deny even the demonstration of His love through the sacrifice of Jesus.

The Jew's refusal to accept Jesus as the anointed one of God, as their Messiah, has cost them a great deal of suffering and pain; it's not that God has caused evil to fall upon them, but that His protection was taken away. They were left exposed to the attacks of God's evil enemy, Satan.

God did not cause the misery that they have suffered. It is a direct consequence of their refusal to accept His anointed. God did not abandon them; they abandoned God by refusing to accept His Son. Had they accepted Jesus at His first coming, they would have been on top of all mankind, and the millenial reign of Christ would have begun then.

However, God knew that they would refuse His anointed and that these attacks would happen. He permitted them, knowing that by them His promises and plan would come to pass.

The attack of the Assyrians scattered the 10 northern Jewish tribes throughout the world with many ending up in Europe and ultimately the New World. Even in the Far East, there are still residual pockets of individuals that practice aspects of Judaism. By the names of many of the Welsh, Spanish, and European descendants, we can see that many have been scattered throughout the New World and are now part of the many nations in these areas.

Many Middle Eastern people are also descendants of Abraham. The all-knowing God promised what He knew would happen, multiplying Abraham's seed as the *"stars of heaven and as the sand which is on the seashore...."*

Chapter 9

1. No other person deified by man, who ever lived, could claim to be _____, but Jesus is recorded in the Bible as being perfect.

2. It would be unacceptable to come for the purpose of _____ God's glory and to dishonor Him with a less than perfect sacrifice.

3. The entire life of Jesus was predestined so that He would fulfill this purpose exactly as God had instructed the Jews to practice for _____ years prior to Jesus.

4. Jesus _____ still the wind, heal the sick, make fine wine from water, multiply bread loafs, raise the dead, and walk on water.

5. He was either who He said He was or He was the greatest _____ to have ever walked the Earth.

6. The Jew's _____ to accept Jesus as the anointed one of God, as their Messiah, has cost them a great deal of suffering and pain; it's not that God has caused evil to fall upon them, but that His protection and guidance was taken away and they were left exposed to the attacks of God's evil enemy, Satan.

Answers: perfect, restoring, 1,500, could, imposter, refusal

Chapter Ten

The Crucifixion

Jesus died a horrible death on what was called a Roman crucifixion just outside the walls of Jerusalem. Few scholars would deny the historical record as recorded in the Gospels and in Josephus' *Antiquities* written in the early '90s C.E.

In an Arabic version of Josephus' testimony of the tenth century found by Professor Shlomo Pines, Josephus offers us an undeniable reference to Jesus: "At this time there was a wise man, who was called Jesus, and his conduct was good, and he was known to be virtuous. And many people from among the Jews and other nations became his disciples. Pilate condemned him to be crucified and to die. They reported that he had appeared to them three days after his crucifixion, and that he was alive. Accordingly, they believed that he was the Messiah, concerning whom the Prophets have recounted wonders." (Josephus, *Antiquities*, 18.63–64)[16]

Paul's testimony of what he received from the apostles – as recorded in 1st Corinthians 15, written just three years after his Damascus experience or five years after Christ's crucifixion and resurrection – documents that the crucifixion and resurrection of Jesus was a well-established fact and affirmed to by the apostles and Jesus' disciples shortly after the actual event took place. This creed establishes what they knew and understood at the time of these events. *"Moreover, brethren, I declare to you the* *gospel which I preached to you, which also you received and in which you stand, by which also you are saved, if you hold fast that word which I preached to you – unless you believed in vain. For I delivered to you first of all that which I also received: that Christ died for our sins according to the Scriptures, and that He was buried, and that He rose again the third day according to the Scriptures, and that He was seen by Cephas, then by the twelve. After that He was seen by over five hundred brethren at once, of whom the greater part remain to the present, but some have fallen asleep. After that He was seen by James then by all the apostles."* (1st Corinthians 15:3–7 NKJV)**

Jesus lived, died by crucifixion, and was resurrected as documented in the aforementioned literary documents. Many arguments are made as to who killed Jesus. Some blame the Jews, and still others blame the Romans. Few understand what Jesus Himself revealed. In the garden when they came to arrest Him, He stated: *"Or do you not think that I cannot now pray to my Father, and He will provide Me with more than twelve legions of angels?"* (Matthew 26:53 NKJV)* And to Pilate, He responded: *"You would have no authority over Me, unless it had been given from above."* (John 19:10–11 NKJV)*

Jesus knew His fate. He repeatedly told His disciples of His approaching death. Had He wanted to get away, He could have done it at any time before His arrest. He gave Himself to be sacrificed because it was the will of the Father. His only reason for living was to do the will of the Father which ought to be our reason for living.

Jesus suffering was in accordance to the prophecies written hundreds of years before Him. His life was not taken from Him. He gave His life up willingly. Blame the Jews, blame the Romans, and blame yourself, for we all took part in killing Jesus. It was for God's purpose. It was our rebellious nature, our sins, for which He died. He died for the purpose of demonstrating to us the love of the Father. This was necessary to fulfill God's plan, to demonstrate His love to us.

The Apostle Peter makes it clear that Jews and Gentiles are responsible for Jesus' crucifixion. *"For truly against Your holy Servant Jesus, whom You anointed, both Herod and Pontius Pilate, with the Gentiles and the people of Israel, were gathered together to do whatever Your hand and Your purpose determined before to be done."* (Acts 4:27–28 NKJV)*

The sacrifice of Christ also provided a means for non-Jews to come to salvation. To the Jews, it was a mystery as to how God was going to save the Gentiles. The mystery of how God would bring His salvation to the non-Jew was revealed by the sacrifice of Christ. God not only revealed how He was going to save the Gentiles through Christ's sacrifice, but in so doing He also revealed to His loyal subjects how He would recoup His glory.

The Church or true believers would be the instruments of this lesson for the principalities and powers in the heavenly places. That is why Paul said: *"To me, who am less than the least of all the saints, this grace was given, that I should preach among the Gentiles the unsearchable riches of Christ, and to make all see what is the fellowship of the mystery, which from the beginning of the ages has been hidden in God who created all things through Jesus Christ; to the intent that now the manifold wisdom of God might be made known by the church to the principalities and powers in the heavenly places, according to the eternal purpose which He accomplished in Christ Jesus our Lord, in whom we have boldness and access with confidence through faith in*

Him. Therefore I ask that you do not lose heart at my tribulations for you, which is your glory." (Ephesians 3:8–13 NKJV)*

Jesus had one great passion, and that passion was to do the will of the Father. Some say His death was nothing worse than the many atrocities we have heard other innocent people suffer. But He suffered voluntarily, and He was no ordinary person. He was not just innocent. He was deity. Worthy of praise, He instead was spat upon, repeatedly punched, kicked and punctured, His skin ripped in hundreds of places by shrapnel-like metal and stone attached to the ends of multiple-stranded whips. His bones separated and His body perforated, He suffered through severe pain, anguish, and thirst. His body was repeatedly brutalized while being scorned and laughed at.

He was treated like no animal should be. But He was not an animal. He was a human being, and not just a human being, but the anointed one of God and the master craftsman in the creation of the universe. For it is written: *"I have been established from everlasting. From the beginning, before there was ever an earth. When there were no depths I was brought forth. When there were no fountains abounding with water, before the mountains were settled, before the hills, I was brought forth; while as yet He had not made the earth or the fields, or the primal dust of the world. When He prepared the heavens, I was there, When He drew a circle on the face of the deep, When He established the clouds above, When He strengthened the fountains of the deep, When He assigned to the sea its limit, So that the waters would not transgress His command, When He marked out the foundations of the earth, Then I was beside Him as a master craftsman; And I was daily His delight, Rejoicing always before Him, Rejoicing in His inhabited* *world, And my delight was with the sons of men." (Proverbs 8:23–31 NKJV)**

This is Jesus, and for this and for who He was, He should have been received with praises and adoration. Yet He was instead received with tortuous evil and hate. His glory was denied, and instead, He was shredded and crucified like a barbarous demon.

There is much discourse about aliens visiting earth and teaching ancient man building techniques and wonders that we today have great difficulty explaining. There are revelations about non-visible constellations and the earth that we have only recently discovered. These revelations have served to establish set times and seasons for humanity. The knowledge of time and seasons has enabled man to integrate God's commands and mandates into their lives. No doubt, it was God's Master Craftsman, His anointed, that made these revelations to humanity, this is why He states, *"Rejoicing in His inhabited world, And my delight was with the sons of men." (Proverbs 8:31 NKJV)** Preparing the way for God's plan."

Chapter 10

1. Jesus died a horrible death on what was called a Roman _____ just outside the walls of Jerusalem.

2. To the _____ it was a mystery as to how God was going to save the Gentiles.

3. God did not only reveal how He was going to save the Gentiles through Christ's sacrifice, but in so doing He also revealed to His loyal subjects how He would _____ His glory.

4. The Church or true believers would be the _____ of this lesson for the principalities and powers in the heavenly places.

5. Jesus had one great passion, and that passion was to do the _____ of the Father.

6. His body was repeatedly _____ while being scorned and laughed at.

Answers: crucifixion, Jews, recoup, instruments, will, brutalized

Chapter Eleven

Abraham's Vision and God's Promise

Jesus proclaimed Himself to be the Son of God. After healing a man who was blind from birth and hearing that this man had been cast out of the synagogue by the Pharisees for stating that *"if this Man (Jesus), were not from God, He could do nothing," (John 9:33 NKJV)** Jesus found him and asked him: *"Do you believe in the Son of God?"* The man answered, *"Who is He, Lord that I may believe in Him?"* and Jesus answered him, *"You have both seen Him and it is He who is talking with you." (John 9:35–37 NKJV)**

The concept of the Son of God was not foreign to the Jews. The book of Proverbs clearly shows that God has a Son for it states: *"Who has ascended into heaven or descended? Who has gathered the wind in His fist? Who has bound the waters in a garment? Who has established all the ends of the earth? What is His name, and what is His Son's name, if you know?" (Proverbs 30:4–5 NKJV)**

This mystery of God's plan with His Son was revealed to Abraham. That is why Jesus could say: *"Abraham saw my day and was glad."* Abraham saw humanity, the lowest of God's creatures, showing up the highest of angels with their love and devotion to the God of the universe. This could only be accomplished through the revelation of God's love through the sacrifice of Jesus' death on the cross.

This was why Abraham was able to consent to giving his son in sacrifice to God because he knew God was willing to give His very own Son for humanity. This was the mission Jesus came to fulfill, and fulfill it He did. We who join Him become His inheritance for a job well done. *"God, who at various times and in various places spoke in times past to the fathers by the prophets, has in these last days spoken to us by His Son, whom He has appointed heir of all things, through whom also he made the worlds; who being the brightness of His glory and the express image of His person, and upholding all things by the word of His power, when He had by Himself purged our sins, sat down at the right hand of the Majesty on high, having become so much better than the angels, as He has by inheritance obtained a more excellent name than they."* (Hebrews 1:1–4 NKJV)*

This was also revealed to King David as he wrote in Psalms 45: *"Your throne, O God, is forever and ever; a scepter of righteousness is the scepter of Your kingdom. You love righteousness and hate wickedness; Therefore God, Your God, has anointed You with the oil of righteousness more than your companions."* (Psalms 45:6–8 NKJV)*

Abraham understood the depth of God's love. He was to be obedient to whatever God asked. God was willing to give His Son. Abraham would have to be willing to give his son to God as well. Having this understanding, Abraham was willing to give God his son Isaac. Isaac also must have understood this great sacrifice. He trusted his father and prepared for the sacrifice, even though it was becoming more apparent to him that he was to be the sacrifice. Isaac by this time was not a young child. Isaac carried the wood and did exactly as his father asked him to do.

When Jesus said that Abraham saw His day and was glad, He was saying that Abraham had revelation of Jesus coming and of the salvation that was coming to the world through Jesus. Abraham saw that his obedience would play a role in God's great plan. For this, Abraham was blessed and his descendants received the promise of greater blessings.

As it is written: *"So Abraham rose early in the morning and saddled his donkey, and took two of his young men with him, and Isaac his son; and he split the wood for the burnt offering, and arose and went to the place of which God had told him. Then on the third day Abraham lifted his eyes and saw the place afar off. And Abraham said to his young men, 'Stay here with the donkey; the lad and I will go yonder and worship and we will come back to you.' So Abraham took the wood of the burnt offering and laid it on Isaac his son; and he took the fire in his hand, and a knife, and the two of them went together. But Isaac spoke to Abraham his father and said, 'My father!' And he said, 'Here I am, my son.' Then he said, 'Look, the fire and the wood, but where is the burnt offering?' And Abraham said, 'My son, God will provide for Himself the lamb for the burnt offering?' So the two of them went together. Then they came to the place of which God had told him. And Abraham built an altar there and placed the wood in order; and he bound Isaac his son and laid him on the altar, upon the wood. And Abraham stretched out his hand and took the knife to slay his son. But the Angel of the Lord called to him from heaven and said, 'Abraham, Abraham!' So he said, 'Here I am.' And He said, 'Do not lay your hand on the lad, or do anything to him; for now I know that you fear God, since you have not withheld your son, your only son, from Me.' Then Abraham lifted his eyes and looked, and there behind him was a ram caught in a thicket by its horns. So Abraham went and took the ram and offered it up for a burnt offering instead of his son. And Abraham called the name of the place, The-Lord-Will-Provide; as it is said to this day, 'In the Mount of the Lord it shall be provided.' Then the Angel of the Lord called to Abraham a second time out of heaven, and said: 'By Myself I have sworn, says the Lord, because you have done this thing, and have not withheld your son, your only son, blessings I will bless you, and multiplying I will multiply your descendants as the stars of the heaven and as the sand which is on the seashore; and your descendants shall possess the gate of their enemies. In your seed all the nations of the earth shall be blessed, because you have obeyed My voice.'"* (Genesis 22:3–18 NKJV)*

That this "seed" refers to Jesus is affirmed in Galatians where it is written: *"Now to Abraham and his seed were the promises made. He does not say 'And to seeds,' as of many, but as of one, 'And to your Seed,' who is Christ."* (Galatians 3:16 NKJV)*

This seed is Jesus, the deliverer of God's promise, through whom the whole world, God's people, could receive salvation. Jesus came as part of God's plan to restore His glory and to build God's Kingdom of perfect and justified individuals. As it is written: *"But you are a chosen generation, a royal priesthood, a holy nation, His own special people, that you may proclaim the praises of Him who called you out of darkness into His marvelous light; who once were not a people but are now the people of God, who had not obtained mercy but now have obtained mercy."* (1 Peter 2:9–10 NKJV)* This passage is specifically speaking of individuals who become a people through their conversion experience, obtaining mercy through Jesus Christ and forming a royal priesthood, a Holy nation, God's own special people. This is not referring to Jews who are and were a people but to Gentiles and Jews who were not a people but become one people through Jesus Christ.

Chapter 11

1. Jesus proclaimed Himself to be the _____ of God.

2. The book of _____ clearly shows that God has a Son.

3. When Jesus said that Abraham saw His day and was glad, He was saying that Abraham had revelation of Jesus coming and of the _____ that was coming to the world through Jesus.

4. For this, Abraham was _____ and his descendants received the promise of greater blessings.

5. Jesus came as part of God's plan to _____ His glory and to build God's Kingdom of perfect and justified individuals.

6. This passage is specifically speaking of individuals who become a people through their _____ experience, obtaining mercy through Jesus Christ and forming a royal priesthood, a Holy nation, God's own special people.

Answers: son, Proverbs, salvation, blessed, restore, conversion

Chapter Twelve

God's Purpose for His Creation

God's purpose in creation is to build a perfect kingdom with loyal and perfect subjects. That is why Jesus, as a man, had to be perfect. We who accept this plan of God and who desire to be a part of His kingdom must become like Jesus in all things, loyal and obedient servants, serving God by serving mankind just as Jesus did.

God does not need our love or our money. He does not even need our adoration. But He enjoys it. Adoration is a way His servants show pleasure with serving Him willingly. The true demonstration of adoration lies in our obedience. We show Him that we love Him by serving and giving to our fellow man, by being honest and sincere, and learning and applying His word, as Jesus did.

Our reward is eternal life. But this does not only entail living eternally in a body such as what we have but a body like the body of the resurrected Jesus, an ideal body. Jesus said: *"Most assuredly, I say to you, he who believes in Me, the works that I do he will do also; and greater works than these he will do, because I go to My Father." (John 14:12 NKJV)**

"Greater works" than the great works and miracles of Jesus is hard to believe. But as believers filled with the Spirit, we should be able to do everything that Christ did and even more. In a glorified body, like the body of the risen Christ, one can only imagine the things we would be able to do. As it is written, *"Beloved, now we are children of God; and it has not yet been revealed what we shall be, but we know that when He is revealed, we shall be like Him, for we shall see Him as He is. And everyone who has this hope in Him purifies himself, just as He is pure."* *(1 John 3:2–3 NKJV)**

The apostle Peter spoke about this inheritance of the believer: *"Blessed be the God and Father of our Lord Jesus Christ, who according to His abundant mercy has begotten us again to a living hope through the resurrection of Jesus Christ from the dead, to an inheritance incorruptible and undefiled and that does not fade away, reserved in heaven for you, who are kept by the power of God through faith for salvation ready to be revealed in the last time."* *(1 Peter 1:3–5 NKJV)** This is the reward for us who choose to accept the sacrifice that Jesus made in dying for our sins, taking on our sins and justifying us before the Father. This has made it possible for us to be transformed into supernatural beings, and not just supernatural beings, but perfected beings before God, like Jesus.

Paul affirms this transformation through Jesus; *"For our citizenship is in heaven, from which we also eagerly wait for the Savior, the Lord Jesus Christ, who will transform our lowly body that it may be conformed to His glorious body, according to the working by which He is able even to subdue all things to Himself."* *(Philippians 3:20-21 NKJV)**

This is the purpose for God's creation, the purpose for our being. From the beginning of time, God saw that rebellion would come and that only by changing the hearts of His subjects through His love could He provide for those that out of their own volition would truly serve Him. They would be His children and He would be their God.

Permitting the rebellious outcast to subsist with His children would serve to separate and to refine and purify His children, just like gems in the raw before their cutting and polishing, thus enhancing their worth.

Paul describes our struggle and our reward when we make the decision to live as the Spirit of God prompts us to, rather than as our evil flesh desires. *"Because the carnal mind is enmity against God; for it is not subject to the law of God, nor indeed can be. So then, those who are in the flesh cannot please God. But you are not in the flesh but in the Spirit, if indeed the Spirit of God dwells in you. Now if anyone does not have the Spirit of Christ, he is not His. And if Christ is in you, the body is dead because of sin, but the Spirit is life because of righteousness. But if the Spirit of Him who raised Jesus from the dead dwells in you, He who raised Christ from the dead will also give life to your mortal bodies through His Spirit who dwells in you."* (Romans 8:7–11 NKJV)* We dwell in the Spirit when we are obedient to God's word and to His desire for our life, constantly mindful of Him and meditating on His word.

Many have not learned this or reject it as nonsense and yet accept the Judeo-Christian Bible as a good moral book. They lose out, not only on the blessings therein but also on the promises of the reward. Some make excuses while others simply refuse to give up their pleasurable sinful ways. These are the choices that God would have us to choose from.

This is exactly what demonstrates our loyalty and love to Him. It demands that we give Him what we prize the most. Like Abraham, we must choose between God and something we have come to love more than ourselves. Only by choosing to sacrifice that which we love for God will God give us the blessings He has in store for us.

God wants us to be like Jesus, putting Him first in all things. We must be obedient to His word and follow the example of His Son Jesus and no one else. Looking to someone who has failed in his walk or to some other god will not excuse you. For through Jesus is the only way that we can please God and receive the reward promised to us — eternal life in a body like Jesus.

Using the excuse that someone who was supposedly following Jesus acted differently or was hypocritical will not excuse anyone since our example is Jesus and no one else. *"For whoever finds Me finds life, and obtains favor from the LORD; but he who sins against Me wrongs his own soul; all those who hate Me love death." (Proverbs 8:35–36 NKJV)**

God's purpose is to build a kingdom of saints, individuals perfected through the refining experience of repenting, accepting God's sacrifice, and converting to a life subservient to Him.

When Jesus was asked what God's greatest commandments were, He responded: *"'You shall love the LORD your God with all your heart, with all your soul, and with all your mind.' This is the first and great commandment. And the second is like it: 'You shall love your neighbor as yourself.' On these two commandments hang all the Law and the Prophets." (Matthew 22:37–40 NKJV)**

This means that you must serve God with your mind, your body, and your money, that is, all that God has given you. Additionally, you must treat others as if they were you, giving to those who are in need whatever is in your power to give.

Sacrificial love is what God wants us to show to others, the same love that Jesus demonstrated on the cross towards each and every one of us. We love not because people deserve it. We love in obedience to God. Love is a fruit that God expects us to produce, and not just by saying it, but by meaning it, showing it with our actions and without regard or reward.

Sacrificial love is what true love is. It is not "what is in it for me," but "how can I serve them." That is how we are to operate with everyone: our wife or husband, our children, our friends, all who we know or meet that has a need. This is how God loves us and is the example of how we are to be to others.

Jesus came on a mission. His mission was to recruit others for God's kingdom. The gift that we receive, or the sign-on bonus that we receive, is eternal life in a perfected body, an ideal body, a body as that of Christ Jesus. With His sacrifice, Christ demonstrated God's love for us in a profound way and showed us how God would have us be to others.

Jesus' attributes are to be our attributes and are to be exhibited as fruits of our conversion. These fruits demonstrate that we have truly become like Jesus. *"But the fruit of the Spirit is love, joy, peace, longsuffering, kindness, goodness, faithfulness, gentleness, self-control. Against such there is no law." (Galatians 5:22 NKJV)**

Demonstrations of the signs of true conversion are "good fruits," changes in our character that make us Christ-like. Changes God requires we make.

While emphasizing that we must bear good fruit, the Bible warns us against those who bear bad fruit and what will happen to those who bear bad fruit. *"Beware of false prophets, who come to you in sheep's clothing, but inwardly* *they are ravenous wolves. You will know them by their fruits. Do men gather grapes from thorn bushes or figs from thistles? Even so, every good tree bears good fruit, but a bad tree bears bad fruit. A good tree cannot bear bad fruit, nor can a bad tree bear good fruit. Every tree that does not bear good fruit is cut down and thrown into the fire. Therefore by their fruits you will know them." (Matthew 7:15–20 NKJV)**

These changes are a demonstration of our commitment to honor the mission that Jesus came to perform. It shows that we have enlisted into the forces which Jesus heads. For this reason, we are called "soldiers of the cross."

Many refuse to embrace the characteristics that God requires of those who are committed to Him. Their commitment is to another way of life. They refuse to change that which they have come to love though it may be detrimental to them. Rather than change for God, they would have God change for them, denying what is in God's Word and making up gods or changing God's Word to fit their lifestyles.

Unfortunately for them, it does not work that way. That is why God is God and we are His servants. What if Abraham had refused to sacrifice his son? Would God have blessed him or his descendants? Actually, God already knew what Abraham would do. The ram was prepared beforehand for Abraham and Isaac's arrival.

Scripture tells us we are to choose between blessings and curses: blessings, if we are obedient; curses, if we refuse to obey. *"Behold, I set before you today a blessing and a curse: the blessing, if you obey the commandments of the LORD your God which I command you today; and the curse, if you do not obey the commandments of the LORD your God, but turn aside from the way which I command you*

today, to go after other gods which you have not known."
(Deuteronomy 11:26–27 NKJV)*

"The blessing" is that He will be with you and give you all that He has promised, and "the curse" is that He will not be with you and ultimately that you will not be with Him. It is your choice. Want to be a part of God's perfect kingdom? Consider your options. Which is more valuable to you? What value would you give for an ideal body that will endure forever?

Is there anything in your life or any amount of money or other possession that could be worth more? *"For what profit is it to a man if he gains the whole world, and loses his own soul? Or what will a man give in exchange for his soul? For the Son of Man will come in the glory of His Father with His angels, and then He will reward each according to his works."* (Matthew 11:26–27 NKJV)*

After the millennial reign of Christ and the end and defeat of Satan, Revelation 21 tells us God's Kingdom, the New Jerusalem, will descend from Heaven and God will dwell with man in a purified new earth.

"Now I saw a new heaven and a new earth, for the first heaven and the first earth had passed away. Also there was no more sea. Then I, John, saw the holy city, New Jerusalem, coming down out of heaven from God, prepared as a bride adorned for her husband. And I heard a loud voice from heaven saying, 'Behold, the tabernacle of God is with men, and He will dwell with them, and they shall be His people. God Himself will be with them and be their God. And God will wipe away every tear from their eyes; there shall be no more death, nor sorrow, nor crying. There shall be no more pain, for the former things have passed away.' Then He who sat on the throne said, 'Behold, I make all things

new.' And He said to me, 'Write, for these words are true and faithful.'" (Revelation 21:1–5 NKJV)*

John describes this incredible city, *"Then one of the seven angels who had the seven bowls filled with the seven last plagues came to me and talked with me, saying, 'Come, I will show you the bride, the Lamb's wife.' And he carried me away in the Spirit to a great and high mountain, and showed me the great city, the holy Jerusalem, descending out of heaven from God, having the glory of God. Her light was like a most precious stone, like a jasper stone, clear as crystal. Also she had a great and high wall with twelve gates, and twelve angels at the gates, and names written on them, which are the names of the twelve tribes of the children of Israel: three gates on the east, three gates on the north, three gates on the south, and three gates on the west. Now the wall of the city had twelve foundations, and on them were the names of the twelve apostles of the Lamb. And he who talked with me had a gold reed to measure the city, its gates, and its wall. The city is laid out as a square; its length is as great as its breadth. And he measured the city with the reed: twelve thousand furlongs. Its length, breadth, and height are equal. Then he measured its wall: one hundred and forty-four cubits, according to the measure of a man, that is, of an angel. The construction of its wall was of jasper; and the city was pure gold, like clear glass. The foundations of the wall of the city were adorned with all kinds of precious stones: the first foundation was jasper, the second sapphire, the third chalcedony, the fourth emerald, the fifth sardonyx, the sixth sardius, the seventh chrysolite, the eighth beryl, the ninth topaz, the tenth chrysoprase, the eleventh jacinth, and the twelfth amethyst. The twelve gates were twelve pearls: each individual gate was of one pearl. And the street of the city was pure gold, like transparent glass. But I saw no temple in it, for the Lord God Almighty* and the Lamb are its temple. The city had no need of the sun or of the moon to shine in it, for the glory of God illuminated it. The Lamb is its light. And the nations of those who are saved shall walk in its light, and the kings of the earth bring their glory and honor into it. Its gates shall not be shut at all by day (there shall be no night there). And they shall bring the glory and the honor of the nations into it. But there shall by no means enter it anything that defiles, or causes an abomination or a lie, but only those who are written in the Lamb's Book of Life."

"Tabernacle" is a term used for the dwelling place of God. In the Bible, it is shown that God in the end will dwell with those who have accepted and have become as His Son, being sanctified through their trials and tribulations.

This New Jerusalem, God's perfect kingdom, coming down from heaven is the finality of God's plan for man. God will tabernacle or dwell with His saints, the perfected ones, who will be His people for ever and ever.

Chapter 12

1. God's purpose in creation is to build a _____ kingdom with loyal and perfect subjects.

2. We, who accept this plan of God and who desire to be a part of His kingdom, must become like Jesus in all things, loyal and obedient servants, serving God by serving _____ just as Jesus did.

3. Demonstrations of the signs of true conversion are "good fruits," changes in our _____ that make us Christ-like.

4. Jesus' attributes are to be our _____ and are to be exhibited as fruits of our conversion.

5. "The blessing" is that He will be with you and give you all that He has promised, and "the curse" is that He will not be with you and _____ that you will not be with Him.

6. Is there anything in your _____ or any amount of money or other possession that could be worth more?

Answers: perfect, mankind, character, attributes, ultimately, life

Chapter Thirteen

Our Shepherd

The LORD is my shepherd;
I shall not want.
He makes me to lie down in green pastures;
He leads me beside the still waters.
He restores my soul;
He leads me in the paths of righteousness
For His name's sake.
Yea, though I walk through the valley of the
shadow of death,
I will fear no evil;
For You are with me;
Your rod and Your staff, they comfort me.
You prepare a table before me in the presence
of my enemies;
You anoint my head with oil;
My cup runs over.
Surely goodness and mercy shall follow me
All the days of my life;
And I will dwell in the house of the LORD
Forever.

(Psalms 23 NKJV)*

In the 23rd Psalm, King David sums up the relationship that we should have with God. In it, he demonstrates that God is our shepherd or caretaker, our restorer, and our rest who leads us in the way of righteousness for His name's sake or for His purpose.

Despite what we may experience, we should not be fearful for He is with us. With His rod, He causes us to move in the direction that He wants us to move in. And with His staff, He keeps us from going in the direction He does not want us to go in, providing us with comfort and assurance. He provides for us even in difficult times and blesses us, assuring us that we will be with Him in His place of dwelling forever.

King David was not perfect. Yet, he was described as the apple of God's eye, implying that God gave David special favor. This is not because David was perfect but because David always earnestly wanted to do right by God, even when he messed up. And because of this, David was assured of eternity. This favor can be ours as well. In Proverbs, it is written: *"Keep my commands and live, And my law as the apple of your eye." (Proverbs 17:2 NKJV)**

God gives us much more than what we give Him. This passage assures us that we too can become the apple of God's eye by being obedient to His word.

God will guide you with His staff, or He will drive you with His rod as long as you will let Him. If you choose to disregard Him, He leaves you alone to your own destruction. *"And even as they did not like to retain God in their knowledge, God gave them over to a debased mind, to do those things which are not fitting; being filled with all unrighteousness, sexual immorality, wickedness,* *covetousness, maliciousness; full of envy, murder, strife, deceit, evil-mindedness; they are whisperers, backbiters, haters of God, violent, proud, boasters, inventors of evil things, disobedient to parents, undiscerning, untrustworthy, unloving, unforgiving, unmerciful; who, knowing the righteous judgment of God, that those who practice such things are deserving of death, not only do the same but also approve of those who practice them." (Romans 1:28–32 NKJV)**

This passage describes the evil times and people that have existed through the ages up to today. We hear individuals living and doing as they like, disregarding that their way of life or that their behavior could be wrong, denying that there is any validity in living as the Scriptures dictate or that there are absolute truths derived from God from which all morality is derived and encouraging others to do the same.

Just as there are absolutes in natural laws, there are absolutes in spiritual laws. And just as there are consequences to not taking into account the natural laws, there are consequences to non-observance of the spiritual laws.

For example, gravity will pull you down to the ground if you jump off of a building just as sure as hate will alter your personality and bring revulsion to your person. This may sound absurd to one who has not dealt in the spiritual, but I have seen this numerous times. That is why the spiritual laws are so powerful and why forgiveness, for example, brings with it so much healing.

For example, take a woman who states: "I will never marry a man like my father because he's a drunkard and beats my mother." What do you think her husband will be like? She has judged her father and violated the fifth commandment of honoring our father and mother and thereby has brought a curse upon herself.

Obedience to God is independent of our relationship to other people or to whether the other person deserves it or not. We obey because we trust God and because we want Him to bless us and because we want to be obedient to Him and to bless Him, that is, to bring goodness to Him as He brings goodness to us.

Jesus advocated forgiveness and love because with forgiveness we receive healing, and with love, we receive love. These do not only change our circumstances, but they also change our inner being, our attitude, and our perception of things. It forms part of our perfection process.

Our healing does not require that the individual who offended us be repentant. They have their own God-given responsibility to repent. If they fail to do so, they will suffer the consequences. We receive healing through forgiveness. Unforgiveness nullifies true repentance and blocks God's blessings and His forgiveness of us.

I can recall an elderly woman who brought her mentally impaired sister into the office for an examination. As I was examining the sister, the elderly woman began to complain of her aching bones and how miserable she felt because of her pain. The complaining was annoying, and not thinking, I turned to her and said, "And who do you hate?"

Without expecting it, she began to sob. I felt remorseful. My intent was not to cause her any grief. My comment was thoughtless, brought on by her complaining. I was repentant and asked her to forgive me, as I explained that the Bible states that "hate rots the bones."

She went on to explain how she hated her daughter because of the way her daughter treated her own children and how her daughter was a bad housekeeper and rude to her when she commented on these things to her.

I went on to explain that there was healing in forgiveness and what she needed to do was to love her daughter even if she did not deserve it. She went on just ranting about what an unloving and hateful person her daughter was. I emphasized to her that regardless of how her daughter was, she was to love her and forgive her, not because she deserved it but because that was what God wanted her to do.

The next morning, this same woman came into my office with a great big smile, thanking me for the advice I had given her. She explained how after leaving the office she went to her daughter's home and asked her daughter to forgive her and told her that she loved her. Her daughter also asked her for forgiveness as well and told her that she loved her too, and they both cried on each other. She commented that that was the best night she had ever spent and that her pains had gone completely away.

There truly is physical healing in forgiveness, as there is illness in hate and envy. The Bible states in Proverbs: *"A sound heart is life to the body, But envy is rottenness to the bones." (Proverbs 14:30 NKJV)**

Sincere forgiveness is a mandate which brings blessings, not to the person who is forgiven, but to the person who does the forgiving.

Repentance by the individual who offended you is not a requirement for your forgiveness of that person.

There is, however, a requirement on the part of the person who offends to repent from his offense for his own healing.

Forgiveness is in fact so important that when Peter asked Jesus how many times he should forgive his brother, Jesus did not answer only once, but seven times seventy: *"Then Peter came to Him and said, 'Lord, how often shall my brother sin against me, and I forgive him? Up to seven times?' Jesus said to him, 'I do not say to you, up to seven times, but up to seventy times seven.'" (Matthew 18:21–22 NKJV)**

Jesus went on to say: *"Therefore, the kingdom of heaven is like a king who wanted to settle accounts with his servants. As he began the settlement, a man who owed him ten thousand talents (~ 89 million denarii) was brought to him. Since he was not able to pay, the master ordered that he and his wife and his children and all that he had be sold to repay the debt. The servant fell on his knees before him. 'Be patient with me,' he begged, 'and I will pay back everything.' The servant's master took pity on him, canceled the debt and let him go. But when that servant went out, he found one of his fellow servants who owed him a hundred denarii. He grabbed him and began to choke him. 'Pay back what you owe me!' He demanded. His fellow servant fell to his knees and begged him, 'be patient with me, and I will pay you back.' But he refused. Instead, he went off and had the man thrown into prison until he could pay the debt. When the other servants saw what had happened, they were greatly distressed and went and told their master everything that had happened. Then the master called the servant in. 'You wicked servant,' he said, 'I canceled all that debt of yours because you begged me to. Shouldn't you have had mercy on your fellow servant just as I had on you?' In anger his master turned him over to the jailers to be tortured, until he should pay back all he owed." (Matthew*

18:23–35 NKJV)* "This is how my heavenly Father will treat each of you unless you forgive your brother from your heart." (Matthew 18:35 NKJV)* He was, in fact, referring to the torture the unforgiving servant was to receive.

The people who offend and do not repent open thenselves up to the wrath of God. This does not mean that God strikes him or her down but that God's protection is taken away from them, and the consequences of their unrepentant life will plague them.

The Bible declares that vengeance is of the Lord. In Romans, Paul writes: *"Beloved, do not avenge yourselves, but rather give place to wrath; for it is written, 'Vengeance is Mine, I will repay,' says the Lord." (Romans 12:19 NKJV)**

In Deuteronomy, it is more explicit. *"Vengeance is Mine, and recompense; their foot shall slip in due time; for the day of their calamity is at hand, and the things to come hasten upon them." (Deuteronomy 32:35 NKJV)**

As a teenager growing up in Brooklyn, New York, I raised pigeons. This was a hobby that I enjoyed. It kept me from getting into trouble.

At one time, I had a pigeon that I kept in our apartment that had never seen the outside of our building. I gave this pigeon away to a friend. He kept his pigeons on the roof of his apartment building. I thought it would be better for my pigeon to be permitted to fly.

Several months later, my friend released the pigeon, and the pigeon flew away. I was very surprised to find this pigeon on the windowsill of our apartment soon after its release. I could never figure out how the pigeon knew the house and the exact apartment where we lived. It was an amazing thing to me, which served to increase my fascination with these birds. Seeing that the birds would return, I put them out on the fire escape of our apartment building and let them out to fly. I only kept a few birds during this time.

On several occasions, two older boys would steal my pigeons. As it was, when the birds were released, they returned to me. Realizing that my pigeons would return to me, the boys on returning, instead of stealing them, would pull their heads off and leave them for me to find. I was devastated. I was unaquainted with these boys, but on learning who they were, my desire was to retaliate against them.

My mother advised me to leave them alone and to secure my birds and let God deal with the boys. I never forgot her words and was reminded of her words when, years later, I learned that one of them was killed when he fell from a twenty-story building onto the concrete pavement below.

The other boy, a young man by this time, had a part of his face and his eye shot out while trying to rob a subway station. God's word, *"Their foot shall slip in due time; For the day of their calamity is at hand, And the things to come hasten upon them,"* (Deuteronomy 32:35 NKJV)* had come to pass.

People who act contrary to God's word think that their actions will go unpunished, but they are only fooling themselves. Whether in this world or in the lake of fire, their recompense will come, and they can be as sure of it as of anything else that they are sure of in their lives.

Unless the individual earnestly repents and transfers their sin to Christ by accepting His sacrifice on the cross, God will not grant them forgiveness and assist them in their restoration. Repentance, acceptance, and forgiveness are key spiritual laws by which we are blessed and receive passage to God's eternal kingdom.

God is particularly protective of His own. Individuals who abuse God's people do not realize the wrath that they expose themselves to. God is more wanting of their repentance, but if repentance does not come; God's protection will not be there when calamity befalls them or their descendants.

God's people are called to pray for them that they may repent and that God be glorified. *"He only is my rock and my salvation; He is my defense; I shall not be greatly moved." (Psalms 62:2 NKJV)**

God's promise is to guide and protect those who trust and obey Him. *"This Book of the Law shall not depart from your mouth, but you shall meditate in it day and night that you may observe to do according to all that is written in it. For then you will make your way prosperous, and then you will have good success. Have I not commanded you? Be strong and of good courage; do not be afraid, nor be dismayed, for the LORD your God is with you wherever you go." (Joshua 1:8–9 NKJV)**

My own experience has shown me God's protection on multiple occasions. At the age of nineteen while returning from a skiing trip in Vermont, heading back to New York on a highway running along a cliff on a winter night, I struck a block of ice that came loose from the car in front of us.

I was traveling with a friend in a front-wheel drive Oldsmobile Starfire. The car went into a spin and struck the snow and ice that was piled up along the railing. The impact caused the car to be flung onto the snow and railing with the rear half of the car hanging over the cliff and the front suspended on the road side of the highway. The fact that the weight was more in the front kept us from going over the clift.

The car was so perfectly balanced on the railing and snow that from the front end we could move the car up and down several inches with one hand. The cliff drop was several hundred feet down. All that could be seen were the lights from the distant houses down below.

Several people stopped and took out shovels from their vehicles and tried to free our vehicle. I was greatly moved by all the kind people who tried to help us.

A tow truck came by and offered to pull us out, but we did not have the money they demanded as payment to get our vehicle pulled. During all the time we were out there, no trucks had gone by.

After a while, when most of the people that had stopped had gone, a man in a Triumph, a small two-passenger sports car, stopped and offered to help us.

To our surprise, this man had a large boat chain in the trunk. He took the chain out and attached it to the bumper of my vehicle and to the frame of his Triumph. Unfortunately, the small Triumph was unable to pull my Oldsmobile Starfire.

The man stepped out of his vehicle and started to disengage the chain, as he said, "Sorry, boys, but I don't think I can help you." I responded, "That's okay; Jesus is with us." The man turned around, surprised by my response, as a fifty-foot semi, the only 18-wheeler that we had seen all the while that we were there, was coming in our direction.

The man began to wave his arms and stopped the semi just a few feet from our vehicle. The truck did not have to back up. The man unhooked the chain from his car and hooked it onto the semi. Within minutes, we were out of there. I was amazed; I knew that because of my relying on Jesus, God had intervened.

As a college student, I drove a yellow taxi cab in New York City from Friday afternoon to Monday morning. I experienced several close calls with attempted holdups and attempts at taking my vehicle. Every one of those times, I would arrive at home and find my mother on her knees praying for my safety. Never did she know what God had saved me from.

I worked until early morning hours in some very dangerous neighborhoods. I was greatly touched by the long hours of prayer my mother undertook for me. It seemed the spirit of God would stir my mother's spirit to pray for me on the days when I was being confronted by one of these situations. I would not tell her the experiences that I had so as not to cause her to worry. Somehow, she knew when I needed prayer the most.

On a July 4th evening, after the fireworks, our family decided to go fishing at the Padre Island pier. On the way to the island, oncoming traffic was very heavy. The two lanes provided no way to pass.

Unaware of a vehicle driving towards us, as the children were singing and discussing the fireworks, I turned around to speak to one of them as our vehicle moved onto the shoulder. The speeding vehicle passed us on our lane, crashing into the vehicle behind us. The drunk driver nearly killed the woman in the vehicle behind us. A head-on crash in our Toyota van would have cost us our lives. I could not understand how we got onto the shoulder but was thankful for God's preservation.

I could remember when our youngest daughter was about two years old. My wife was alone with her when a woman from the neighborhood came by to pick up some clothes for the church. Our daughter was asleep in the house while my wife was talking and helping the woman put the boxes of clothes into her vehicle. Our daughter got up and wandered outside without my wife noticing her.

Our home is surrounded by oxbow lakes — finger tributaries from the Rio Grande — now used for flood control. They are called *resacas*. These *resacas* look like rivers and have rocks and dirt banks which are quite slippery, and we had no fences around the house to keep anyone from wandering into them at the time.

When my wife finished helping the neighbor, she went inside to check on our daughter. She could not find her and realized that she had left the door open. She became frantic and raced outside, looking for our daughter around the house.

Our daughter suddenly appeared, soaking wet, covered with mud from head to toe in the very place where the neighbor's vehicle had been parked. There was no trail of water to indicate how our daughter had gotten there. To this day, we cannot explain what happened or how our daughter got to where she was in the condition that she was in.

Living in obedience to God's Word and in compliance to God's spiritual laws is a means of self and family preservation. This is not to be an occasional practice but a way of life, the goal of which is to please Him who paid for us with His blood.

There are many spiritual laws that apply to our daily lives that help us to be transformed into the person God would have us become, that is, like Christ Jesus. These laws are not only of benefit in our molding process but also help us in our physical preservation and serve as blessings to those who obey and live by them.

Aside from the laws that govern our attitude, such as the requirement to love and rejoice in all things, there are the laws dealing with God's commands. For example, honoring your mother and father is a command that extends our physical life. *"Honor your father and your mother, so that you may live long in the land the LORD your God is giving." (Exodus 20:12 NKJV)**

It is not enough that we love them. If we say we do, we must also honor and respect them, that is, to esteem them highly. This does not require that they deserve it. We love them, despite what they may deserve in obedience to God's word. In so doing, we are blessed.

A friend was in one of these situations. Her father had abandoned their family when she was a little girl. He had another family and did not try to reconcile with his children even after they were grown. She would see him around town but would ignore him.

One day, while discussing problems that she was having with her son, she told me about her father and how they avoided each other. I told her that that was a curse that she had to break, as it would affect her own children. Later on, I learned that she had taken my advice and had initiated to reconcile with her father.

Within a year of their reconciliation, her father unexpectedly died and she was able to go and take her children to pay their last respects to their grandfather at his funeral. She was grateful for my advice for she did not have to deal with any regrets and now had a much larger family than she had before.

I could see that God was guiding her in her walk. He used me to save her from the grief of guilt and the curse of unforgiveness. God blessed her for her obedience.

God wants obedience from us more than sacrifices, as written in 1st Samuel: *"Has the LORD as great delight in burnt offerings and sacrifices, as in obeying the voice of the LORD? Behold, to obey is better than sacrifice, And to heed than the fat of rams. For rebellion is as the sin of witchcraft, and stubbornness, is as iniquity and idolatry. Because you have rejected the word of the LORD, He also has rejected you ...."* (1 Samuel 15:22–23 NKJV)*

God gives up on people who refuse to listen to Him after so many attempts. God gives them up to a debased or reprobate mind.

Do you have a debased or reprobate mind? Do you argue about the existence of God? Do you refuse to hear anything about God or refuse to change a destructive way of life? Do you feel God has given up on you? The wonderful thing is that it is never too late. As long as you have life, you have a chance, regardless of what you have done or of your age.

In Ephesians, Paul writes: *"But God, who is rich in mercy, because of His great love with which He loved us, even when we were dead in trespasses, made us alive together with Christ (by grace you have been saved), and raised us up together, and made us sit together in the heavenly places in Christ Jesus, that in the ages to come He might show the exceeding riches of His grace in His kindness toward us in Christ Jesus. For by grace you have been saved through faith, and that not of yourselves; it is the gift of God, not of works, lest anyone should boast. For we are His workmanship, created in Christ Jesus for good works, which God prepared beforehand that we should walk in them."* (Ephesians 2:4–10 NKJV)**

There is no chance after death. Your decision must be made before death. There is no place of cleansing after death spoken of in the Judeo-Christian Bible as some may believe. And you cannot earn it by being good. God's standard is perfection, and we are all imperfect. And it's not by good works because we were made to do good as it states: *"For we are His workmanship, created in Christ Jesus for good works, which God prepared beforehand that we should walk in them."* (Ephesians 2:10 NKJV)**

Some people come to accept Christ as a medium for their preservation. They are financially strapped or about to suffer great loss or have a terminal disease or a relative or loved one with a terminal disease. They give in to God as their last hope. Their faith is temporal. If not for their problem, they would not be seeking God. Oftentimes, their observance is superficial. They continue to seek and even pleasure in their old ways yet acknowledging that it is against the will of Him from whom they are seeking an answer to their problem. God is not fooled. Like God told Abraham, He tells them to give Him their most prized possession, their lives, their child's life, or whatever that may be. Submission must be complete. You want your life? You must be willing to give Him your life.

God is not a medium; He is God, and He will not let Himself be used as a medium. In fact, He hates mediums and witchcraft. *"There shall not be found among you anyone who makes his son or his daughter pass through the fire, or one who practices witchcraft, or a soothsayer, or one who interprets omens, or a sorcerer, or one who conjures spells, or a medium, or a spiritist, or one who calls up the dead. For all who do these things are an abomination to the LORD, and because of these abominations the LORD your God drives them out from before you." (Deuteronomy 18:10–12 NKJV)**

Will people who accept Jesus as their Lord and Savior gain salvation and enter God's eternal kingdom though they were not fully committed or came to salvation's grace on their deathbed and never really had an opportunity to demonstrate their commitment? This is a question which many people ponder since so many come to know Christ so late in life, or on the verge of death, and do not have an opportunity to demonstrate their faith.

We know that last minute conversions result in salvation. Our example is the criminal who was crucified with Christ. This man acknowledged that Jesus was the anointed one of God the Father and in so doing was given the promise of paradise after death. *"There were also two others, criminals, led with Him to be put to death. And when they had come to the place called Calvary, there they crucified Him, and the criminals, one on the right hand and the other on the left. Then Jesus said, 'Father, forgive them,* for they do not know what they do.' And they divided His garments and cast lots. And the people stood looking on. But even the rulers with them sneered, saying, 'He saved others; let Him save Himself if He is the Christ, the chosen of God.' The soldiers also mocked Him, coming and offering Him sour wine, and saying, 'If You are the King of the Jews, save Yourself.' And an inscription also was written over Him in letters of Greek, Latin, and Hebrew: THIS IS THE KING OF THE JEWS. Then one of the criminals who were hanged blasphemed Him, saying, 'If You are the Christ, save Yourself and us.' But the other, answering, rebuked him, saying, 'Do you not even fear God, seeing you are under the same condemnation? And we indeed justly, for we receive the due reward of our deeds; but this Man has done nothing wrong.' Then he said to Jesus, 'Lord, remember me when You come into Your kingdom.' And Jesus said to him, 'Assuredly, I say to you, today you will be with Me in Paradise.'" (Luke 23:32-43 NKJV)*

It is my opinion that the reason for the 1,000-year reign of Christ after His second coming is due to so many making it by the skin of their teeth. That is, they will only have the bare minimum of what God wants for their salvation, acceptance of Christ and of His sacrifice.

While many religions add additional requirements for salvation, God's mercy is as unfathomable as His great and awesome power. Those who make it will be given additional opportunities to demonstrate their loyalty and dedication to Christ during the 1,000-year reign. Those who fail and reject Christ will be condemned to the great lake of fire in which Satan and his demons will be cast into. This is called the second death. "He who has an ear, let him hear what the Spirit says to the churches. He who overcomes shall not be hurt by the second death." (Revelation 2:11 NKJV)*

When we repent and accept the sacrifice that Jesus Christ made for us and commit to following and becoming like Him, we receive justification, forgiveness of our sins, and at His return, the transformation to perfection that will enable us to reside in God's perfect Kingdom. By accepting God's sacrifice, we become eligible for God's holy nation. *"But you are a chosen generation, a royal priesthood, a holy nation, His own special people, that you may proclaim the praises of Him who called you out of darkness into His marvelous light; who once were not a people but are now the people of God, who had not obtained mercy but now have obtained mercy." (1 Peter 2:9–10 NKJV)**

God gives His promises to you by grace, that is, something you do not deserve. God makes you a candidate of His eternal kingdom because of His mercy and love and not because you deserve it, because no one does. This permits God's Spirit to begin working in you, changing the very substance of your being, renewing and transforming your mind. *"I beseech you therefore, brethren, by the mercies of God, that you present your bodies a living sacrifice, holy, acceptable to God, which is your reasonable service. And do not be conformed to this world, but be transformed by the renewing of your mind, that you may prove what is that good and acceptable and perfect will of God." (Romans 12:1–2 NKJV)**

I have heard individuals in the past confess that God could not forgive them for what they have done. The wonderful thing about the God of the Bible is His mercy. When Christ came, He showed us not only the greatness of God's love but also the greatness of His mercy. What mankind did in crucifying God's Son was deserving of annihilation, yet God through it all showed us how merciful He was.

In the Bible, there are various tales of God's mercy. The story of David and his adulterous relationship with Bathsheba is one such story. David had Uriah, Bathsheba's husband, killed so he could have Bathsheba. *"It happened in the spring of the year, at the time when kings go out to battle, that David sent Joab and his servants with him, and all Israel; and they destroyed the people of Ammon and besieged Rabbah. But David remained at Jerusalem. Then it happened one evening that David arose from his bed and walked on the roof of the king's house. And from the roof he saw a woman bathing, and the woman was very beautiful to behold. So David sent and inquired about the woman. And someone said, 'Is this not Bathsheba, the daughter of Eliam, the wife of Uriah the Hittite?' Then David sent messengers, and took her; and she came to him, and he lay with her, for she was cleansed from her impurity; and she returned to her house. And the woman conceived; so she sent and told David, and said, 'I am with child.' Then David sent to Joab, saying, 'Send me Uriah the Hittite.' And Joab sent Uriah to David. When Uriah had come to him, David asked how Joab was doing, and how the people were doing, and how the war prospered. And David said to Uriah, 'Go down to your house and wash your feet.' So Uriah departed from the king's house, and a gift of food from the king followed him. But Uriah slept at the door of the king's house with all the servants of his lord, and did not go down to his house. So when they told David, saying, 'Uriah did not go down to his house,' David said to Uriah, 'Did you not come from a journey? Why did you not go down to your house?' And Uriah said to David, 'The ark and Israel and Judah are dwelling in tents, and my lord Joab and the servants of my lord are encamped in the open fields. Shall I then go to my house to eat and drink, and to lie with my wife? As you live, and as your soul lives, I will not do this thing.' Then David said to Uriah, 'Wait here today also, and tomorrow I will let* you depart.' So Uriah remained in Jerusalem that day and the next. Now when David called him, he ate and drank before him; and he made him drunk. And at evening he went out to lie on his bed with the servants of his lord, but he did not go down to his house. In the morning it happened that David wrote a letter to Joab and sent it by the hand of Uriah. And he wrote in the letter, saying, 'Set Uriah in the forefront of the hottest battle, and retreat from him, that he may be struck down and die.' So it was, while Joab besieged the city, that he assigned Uriah to a place where he knew there were valiant men. Then the men of the city came out and fought with Joab. And some of the people of the servants of David fell; and Uriah the Hittite died also. Then Joab sent and told David all the things concerning the war, and charged the messenger, saying, 'When you have finished telling the matters of the war to the king, if it happens that the king's wrath rises, and he says to you: "Why did you approach so near to the city when you fought? Did you not know that they would shoot from the wall? Who struck Abimelech the son of Jerubbesheth? Was it not a woman who cast a piece of a millstone on him from the wall, so that he died in Thebez? Why did you go near the wall?" – then you shall say, 'Your servant Uriah the Hittite is dead also.' So the messenger went, and came and told David all that Joab had sent by him. And the messenger said to David, 'Surely the men prevailed against us and came out to us in the field; then we drove them back as far as the entrance of the gate. The archers shot from the wall at your servants; and some of the king's servants are dead, and your servant Uriah the Hittite is dead also.' Then David said to the messenger, 'Thus you shall say to Joab: "Do not let this thing displease you, for the sword devours one as well as another. Strengthen your attack against the city, and overthrow it." So encourage him.' When the wife of Uriah heard that Uriah her husband was dead, she mourned for her husband. And when her mourning was over, David sent and brought her to his house, and she became his wife and bore him a son. But the thing that David had done displeased the LORD." (2 Samuel 11:1–27 NKJV)*

Uriah was a loyal and honorable servant who could not see himself sleeping in a comfortable bed with his wife while his fellow soldiers and brothers and the Ark of God dwelt in tents. When David saw that he could not break Uriah's loyalty, he had him killed. This was a despicable act by a man who claimed to be seeking after God.

God then sent the prophet Nathan to David. David was convicted, but because he repented, God had mercy on him and did not kill him, as David would have done had he been God. But the event was not without consequences since it cost David his son. *"Then the LORD sent Nathan to David. And he came to him, and said to him: 'There were two men in one city, one rich and the other poor. The rich man had exceedingly many flocks and herds. But the poor man had nothing, except one little ewe lamb which he had bought and nourished; and it grew up together with him and with his children. It ate of his own food and drank from his own cup and lay in his bosom; and it was like a daughter to him. And a traveler came to the rich man, who refused to take from his own flock and from his own herd to prepare one for the wayfaring man who had come to him; but he took the poor man's lamb and prepared it for the man who had come to him.' So David's anger was greatly aroused against the man, and he said to Nathan, 'As the LORD lives, the man who has done this shall surely die! And he shall restore fourfold for the lamb, because he did this thing and because he had no pity.' Then Nathan said to David, 'You are the man! Thus says the LORD God of Israel: "I anointed you king over Israel, and I delivered you from the hand of Saul. I gave you your master's house and your master's wives into* *your keeping, and gave you the house of Israel and Judah. And if that had been too little, I also would have given you much more! Why have you despised the commandment of the LORD, to do evil in His sight? You have killed Uriah the Hittite with the sword; you have taken his wife to be your wife, and have killed him with the sword of the people of Ammon. Now therefore, the sword shall never depart from your house, because you have despised Me, and have taken the wife of Uriah the Hittite to be your wife" Thus says the LORD: "Behold, I will raise up adversity against you from your own house; and I will take your wives before your eyes and give them to your neighbor, and he shall lie with your wives in the sight of this sun. For you did it secretly, but I will do this thing before all Israel, before the sun." So David said to Nathan, 'I have sinned against the LORD.' And Nathan said to David, 'The LORD also has put away your sin; you shall not die. However, because by this deed you have given great occasion to the enemies of the LORD to blaspheme, the child also who is born to you shall surely die.'" (2 Samuel 12:1–14 NKJV)**

God forgave David, but there were consequences to his disobedience. If God could forgive such atrocious actions by one of His own, He could easily forgive the offenses of one who is not a follower but who desires to be. This is the beauty of our merciful God.

I would like to bring out another point at this time which I feel is important for the perfecting process of loyal men like Uriah. Uriah was a good servant and a loyal soldier, but he obviously was not a very good husband. This probably contributed to Bathsheba's unfaithfulness, though David, as king, had undue influence over her.

In Judaism during ancient times, the laws of purity and impurity (tumah and taharah) were much more practiced than they are today. An individual was considered ritually impure when he had contact with the dead, loss of menstrual blood, loss of semen due to a wet dream, leprosy, or contact with someone or something which was ritually impure. Immersion in the waters of the mikveh, a pool containing water derived from a natural source, provided a means of transforming the individual, male or female, from a state of ritual impurity to a state of purity.

The laws of niddah prescribe the ritual status of a menstruating woman and her participation in sex, derived from God's commandments in the book of Leviticus, which declares that a woman is ritually impure during her menstrual flow and for seven days afterwards, during which time sexual contact is forbidden. *"When she is cleansed from her discharge, she must count off seven days, and after that she will be ceremonially clean." (Leviticus 15:28 NKJV)**

The period of impurity and waiting puts a woman at risk of pregnancy, as she is poised to be ovulating about the time that she is ceremonially clean. No doubt God caused this to come about so that His people would be fruitful as He desired them to be. Back then, only the God who created us would know when a woman would be ovulating.

A woman takes her ritual bath on the eighth day. After her ceremonial bath, she is able to be with her husband. Bathsheba was taking her ritual bath when she was seen by King David. This implies that she was preparing for Uriah's return and was expecting Uriah to return any day.

Uriah, instead of sleeping at home, decided to sup-port his buddies, thus devaluing his wife who had been making preparations for his return. No doubt, this was a troubled marriage. A woman who has little contact with the outside gets a major share of her self-esteem from her husband. No doubt, this attractive woman was not made to feel attractive by her husband. She was susceptible to the advances of King David, a handsome man and a powerful king.

The failure to appreciate adequately and show value and honor to one's spouse and children is a common flaw among many men, especially men of the faith. Many justify their behavior by claiming they are doing God's work or working to maintain the family. They forget that the family needs more than just what could be purchased. They need his interaction with them. Neglect by the father in pastoral homes is so common that being a pastor's son is an acceptable excuse for being a renegade.

Ministers need to understand that their first and foremost ministry is at home. We do not give enough positive strokes and attention to the people whom we should value the most. They need it, and we need it. Plus, we could be influencing them in their decision-making when they are confronted with a decision which may greatly affect their own lives.

Speaking on transformation, a member of the body that we must learn to train is the tongue. The Bible tells us that the power of life and death is in the tongue. *"Death and life are in the power of the tongue, And those who love it will eat its fruit." (Proverbs 18:21 NKJV)**

If we say we love God, then only things that edify, that is, things that build a person up should come out of our mouths. Words such as "you are good for nothing" or "you will never amount to much," or "I hate you" or other hurtful words said to cause pain or to show rejection or displeasure should never come out of our mouths.

Many times, such words are used in fits of anger or intentionally to inflict pain. Such words, however, can have long term effects, especially when used on impressionable children.

I can recall a ten year old child who was brought to me by his mother. The mother entered his room while he was trying to hang himself.

His parents had broken up several weeks earlier, and the boy, wanting to see his father, went to his place of employment. The father became enraged and told him he was not his son and that he did not love him and chased him away while beating him so he would leave. The boy went back home crying.

The mother assured me that the man was the boy's natural father. That they were having financial problems and that she did not know why he had treated his son that way.

The boy was having a very difficult time with the rejection, at times crying uncontrollably. His school work had deteriorated, and he was becoming a behavioral problem. On that day, the mother walked into his room and found him with a rope around his neck trying to hang himself from the ceiling fan.

I spent a long time counselling the boy and trying to lift him up, telling him about Father God's love and how special he was and making up excuses for his father's behavior.

This may sound like something that rarely occurs, but in actuality, it is a frequent occurrence. Most people have no idea how damaging their words are. There truly is life and death in the tongue. We should gauge every word that we speak so that we not damage but help those we know to grow.

We should address everyone, especially our family with loving and edifying words. We will be better for it, but best of all; we will be helping to build them up.

Chapter 13

1. God will guide you with His staff, or He will drive you with His _____ as long as you will let Him.

2. Living in obedience to God's Word and in compliance to God's spiritual laws is a means of self and family _____.

3. God is not fooled. Like God told Abraham, God tells them to give Him their most _____ possession, their lives, their child's life, or whatever that may be.

4. God gives His promises to you by _____, that is, something you do not deserve but that God gives to you because of His mercy and love.

5. If God could forgive such _____ actions by one of His own, He could easily forgive the offenses of one who is not a follower but who desires to be.

6. Immersion in the waters of the _____, a pool containing water derived from a natural source, provided a means of transforming the individual, male or female, from a state of ritual impurity to a state of purity.

Answers: rod, preservation, prized, grace, atrocious, mikveh

Chapter Fourteen

The Ideal Church Body

The church is not a building but a people. The church is the body of Christ, a body of people. Today, with so many religions and so many practices and traditions, it is confusing as to which one is correct and which one an individual should follow.

I do not know of a perfect religion, and I wonder if Jesus Christ were to return today where He would go to worship. Would He go to a synagogue, or would He go to a Christian church? Certainly, the fact that the Jews did not accept Him did not keep Him from going to the temple. Would the fact that there are so many pagan practices in Christian institutions keep Christ from these institutions?

None of the customary practices that Jesus would have encountered in the temple of His time are being practiced in Christian churches today. Messianic congregations, which blend Christian and Jewish practices, would probably be more acceptable. But should not all be doing the same thing? Why aren't they?

If Christians had obeyed Paul and followed the Old Testament teachings as they were advised to do, *"All Scripture (referring to the Old Testament) is given by inspiration of God, and is profitable for doctrine, for reproof, for correction, for instruction in righteousness,"* (2 Timothy 3:16)*;*"Now I praise you, brethren, that you remember me in all things and keep the traditions just as I delivered them to you."(1 Corinthians 1:2 NKJV)** And kept the feast, there would not be the many denominational differences that exist today. These differences have brought curses and division to God's people.

Regardless of your religious affiliation, the practices of your congregation are very different from what Jesus Christ would have encountered in the temple. Still, each faith ridicules the other as being wrong and being lost. Has God failed? Are all lost though they tried to follow Jesus? Has man made a mockery out of God? Or has Satan made a mockery out of man? If the churches are following Jesus, where is their love for one another and why aren't they honoring the Holy Convocations mandated by God?

Paul advises in his letter to the Galatians: *"Now the works of the flesh are evident, which are: adultery, fornication, uncleanness, lewdness, idolatry, sorcery, hatred, contentions, jealousies, outbursts of wrath, selfish ambitions, dissensions, heresies, envy, murders, drunkenness, revelries, and the like; of which I tell you beforehand, just as I also told you in time past, that those who practice such things will not inherit the kingdom of God."* (Galatians 5:19–20 NKJV)* These are recognized collectively as sin. Anyone desiring to please God would not practice sin. Still many are not in compliance.

I want; however, to talk specifically about one sin in particular, one that appears to be disregarded by the church as a whole, and that is heresy. Heresy is the choosing and holding of an opinion, belief, tradition, or practice that is in conflict with God's Word, that is, choosing to do differently than what God's Word would have us do.

Since Paul wrote this in the first century, it refers to practices and customs contained in the Hebrew Bible since the New Testament did not yet exist.

All of the practices of Jesus were in line with the Jewish Bible since He was a Jew and adhered to the practices and customs of His people. Heresy, then, is choosing and holding of an opinion, belief, and tradition or practice that is in conflict with the Hebrew Bible.

When we look at heresy from this perspective, many of the practices and customs in current Christian congregations are out of compliance with the Hebrew Old Testament.

Many of our current practices and celebrations are primarily derived from pagan traditions or a mingling of pagan and Biblical traditions. Some examples are the observation of Easter, Christmas, and the Communion during mass which uses the round Eucharist, which at one time was used by the pagans and was symbolic of the sun god.

The bread in the Hebrew tradition is symbolic of God's sustenance, a reminder that we are to depend on God for everything. Christ referred to this sustaining power of God as His body, confirming that it was referring to Him who was to become a part of us.

Christmas has a strong resemblance to an early Babylonian custom practiced during the winter solstice (shortest day of the year in late December) in which a tree is adorned and gifts placed on it as an offering to the sun god Tammuz or Nimrod. The large shiny balls are symbolic of the sun.

God's word warns against this practice: *"Thus says the LORD: 'Do not learn the way of the Gentiles; Do not be dismayed at the signs of heaven, For the Gentiles are dismayed at them. For the customs of the peoples are futile;*

For one cuts a tree from the forest, The work of the hands of the workman, with the ax. They decorate it with silver and gold; They fasten it with nails and hammers So that it will not topple. They are upright, like a palm tree, And they cannot speak; They must be carried, Because they cannot go by themselves. Do not be afraid of them, For they cannot do evil, Nor can they do any good.'" (Jeremiah 10:2–5 NKJV)*

Regardless of the arguments as to its derivation, Easter should be a Passover celebration. No amount of argument can justify Easter eggs and many of the practices that have evolved in association with it. Most Christians do not know that the last supper which we commemorate with the Holy Communion actually occurred on the Day of Preparation for the Passover.

The Passover occurred on the day in which Jesus was crucified. Jesus was God's beloved Passover lamb, His most treasured possession. The sacrifice of Jesus was a demonstration of God's profound love for us.

Few individuals in Christian churches know or understand much of the meaning and purposes of the holy convocations or that the first-century Christians were considered a sect of Jews. In fact, many of the Jewish sects in the first century were believers in Jesus as their Messiah. Josephus in his writings attested to the fact that many of the Jews were disciples of Jesus. "And many people from among the Jews and other nations became his disciples."[17]

The Zealots, who overthrew the Herodians prior to the Romans destroying ancient Jerusalem in 70 AD, were believers. They came against the Herodians after one of the temple priests pushed James, who was their high priest and a step-brother of Jesus, off the pinnacle of the temple for preaching Jesus. Our early Christian fathers were considered

Jews and practiced Jewish traditions of worship and the Feast.[18]

The holy convocations are not only prophetic events and memorials of the Jewish experience but also of the Christian walk. For example, the Passover with its related celebrations of Unleavened Bread and First Fruits represents the Christian conversion or coming out of sin, symbolized by the Jews coming out of Egypt.

The Unleavened Bread represents the purification or the putting off of leaven which is representative of putting sin out of our lives. This is symbolized by the Jews removing the leaven from their homes.

The First Fruits represents the resurrection with Christ being the first. This is symbolized by the first harvest of crops by the Jews.

The Pentecost is a memorial for the giving of the Ten Commandments to the Jew and the arrival of the Holy Spirit to the Christian. The two events should be of great significance to the Christian. Still many Christians do not know that the Pentecost also commemorates the giving of the Ten Commandments by God. (Exodus 19)

The related celebrations of Feast of Trumpets, Day of Atonement, and Feast of Tabernacles represent a Christian's preparation or call to worship, as it does for Jews, symbolizing the purification of the church and the arrival and coming again of the Messiah. The Christian's preparation involves getting equipped through the donning of Christian values and strengths described as the armor of God.

The Day of Atonement was the day the high priest would go before the Holy of Holies to ask for forgiveness for the people. This is representative of the sacrifice of Christ on the cross and God's dispensing of forgiveness to all sinners. On this day, Jews have to forgive anyone who has offended them and ask for forgiveness for any offenses they may have committed in line with the repentance required of Christians.

The Feast of Tabernacles commemorates the Jews' travels in the wilderness after leaving Egypt. During this feast, they build sparsely covered booths exposing the outdoors and sky to remind them of the time their ancestors spent in the desert. This is also symbolic of the vulnerability of the Jew and Christian and their need to rely on the creator of the universe. This is answered by the arrival of their redeemer Christ who is believed to have been born during Tabernacles. The ancient prophesy of the return of Elijah during Passover, occurred during the birth of John the Baptist who was six months older than Jesus.

The birth of John was pronounced as the birth of the spirit of Elijah to Zechariah, John's father, by the angel Gabriel. *"Then an angel of the Lord appeared to Zechariah. The angel was standing at the right side of the incense altar. When Zechariah saw him, he was amazed and terrified. But the angel said to him, "Do not be afraid, Zechariah. Your prayer has been heard. Your wife Elizabeth will have a child. It will be a boy, and you must name him John. He will be a joy and delight to you. His birth will make many people very glad. He will be important in the Lord's eyes. "He must never use wine or other such drinks. He will be filled with the Holy Spirit from the time he is born. He will bring many of Israel's people back to the Lord their God. And he will prepare the way for the Lord. He will have the same spirit and power that Elijah had. He will teach parents how to love their* *children. He will also teach people who don't obey to be wise and do what is right. In this way, he will prepare a people who are ready for the Lord." (Luke 1:11-17 NKJV)**

Six months after Passoveer would put Jesus' birth during Tabernacles. The shepherds being out in the fields when the angels announced Christ's birth indicates the Feast of Tabernacles being practiced at the time of the angel's pronouncement of Christ's birth.

During the night, the sheep would be in their pens and not out in the fields, except during the feast of Tabernacles: *"Now there were in the same country shepherds living out in the fields, keeping watch over their flock by night. And behold, an angel of the Lord stood before them, and the glory of the Lord shone around them, and they were greatly afraid. Then the angel said to them, 'Do not be afraid, for behold, I bring you good tidings of great joy which will be to all people. For there is born to you this day in the city of David a Savior, who is Christ the Lord. And this will be the sign to you: You will find a Babe wrapped in swaddling cloths, lying in a manger.' And suddenly there was with the angel a multitude of the heavenly host praising God and saying: 'Glory to God in the highest, And on earth peace, goodwill toward men.'" (Luke 2:8–14 NKJV)**

The preparation for the feasts involves many people and takes much time. It is obvious that God wants His people busy doing His work. We have been deceived into believing that all He wants us to do is to warm pews a couple of hours a week. If anything, celebrating the feast teaches a person how committed God wants his people to be.

Each one of us needs to assess our practices and decide for ourselves what practice would please God and better prepare us for God's coming kingdom. This is important since Paul warns us that "those who practice such things (heresy) will not inherit the Kingdom of God."

Many faiths snub their noses at the practices of other believers. Some argue that Jesus' real name is not Jesus but Yeshua, Yehoshua, Yehushua, Yehusha, or whatever other pronunciation they wish to use. The name "Jesus" is an English translation of the Greek word `Iesou (Ἰησοῦς). This Greek word is a transliteration of the Hebrew word "salvation" which some say is "Yeshua."

Others argue that the "J" does not exist in Hebrew and that the name "Jesus" is not truly representative of the name of the son of God and that we should be using His Hebrew name.

Another argument is that Yeshu means illegitimate in Hebrew. The proper pronunciation is "Yashua" as when pronouncing the "Yah" in Yahveh the Father. As is written, "...My name shall be in Him." (Exodus 23:21 NKJV)* Hence, "Yeh" would not be appropriate and it would have to be "Yah."

Some use "Yahushua," possibly representative of "yah-hat-zil" or "yah-yaw-shah" – "יהוה הציל" – interpreted as meaning Yahveh saves. Others feel that this is more representative of Joshua more so than of Jesus which should be "Yahveh's salvation" or "Yah-shua," meaning "salvation."

Whether you use Jesus, Yashua, Yahushua, or just Yah, God knows the heart, and it is the heart by which our intentions are measured. There have been many miracles using the name of "Jesus"; thus, it's been shown that God aproves of the name and is merciful toward our ignorance.

The proper best pronunciation is probably "Yah-shua." "Yahushua" which represents "Yahveh saves" can also be used since it is the "Yah" which actually refers to the name of God.

There is no consensus on how the Hebrew name of Jesus should be pronounced, but we should never use or pronounce Jesus' Hebrew name as Yeshu since His name is the same as that of the Father "Yahveh" or "Yah."

Yahveh is written as "Yahweh" in English and represents the Tetragrammaton, the letters that represent the name of God "יהוה". These letters are "י" YOD, "ה" HE, "ו" VAV, "ה" HE. The last sylabus therefore should be pronounced as with a "V" and not a "W" as in Yahveh. Jesus said in John 5:43 "I have come in My Father's name...."; hence, we encompass the Godhead when we say Yah.

The word hallelujah or "halleluyah" means "Praise be to God" or "Hale be to Yah" – "Yah" being "Yah" the Father and "Yah" the Son. Being that they have the same name, we praise the Father and the Son when we say hallelujah that is, pronouncing the "j" as a "y" as in "Yah."

It is important that we pronounce God's name and Jesus name correctly, since the Bible teaches us that there is power in the name, " *And whatever you ask in My name, that I will do, that the Father may be glorified in the Son. If you ask anything in My name, I will do it.*" (John 14:13 NKJV)* – Your best bet then is to use "Yah" since we know that hallelujah is the same in all languages and the last part of hallelujah is God's name "Yah." It has not changed despite the years, cultures, or languages that it has been filtered through. Personally, I prefer "Yahshua" and believe that this is the proper way to pronounce it.

It is important that we know and understand God's word. We cannot do or be what He wants if we do not have knowledge of God's word.

There are some who worship their religion and not God and could care less about these issues. They refuse to hear anything except what they have come to accept, trusting not in God but in the dogma of their religion. They claim that they have the truth without knowing the truth. They argue anyone who refuses to accept their way is lost and their worship worthless. We need to remember Paul's warning, *"But even if we, or an angel from heaven, preach any other gospel to you than what we have preached to you, let him be accursed. "* (Galatians 1:8 NKJV)*

We must base our beliefs on God's word and not on some religious dogma. Religious dogma that does not agree with God's word must be discarded. We must, however, be open-minded and willing to search and to verify lest we be wrong.

Some folks hate other people and still expect to make it to God's holy kingdom. They are unwilling to change their attitude and yet expect to be admitted to God's holy kingdom, expecting that the other party does not make it.

There are others who take pride in being obnoxious and contrary. They do not seem to care who they offend and forget that the characteristics of Jesus are to be exhibited in their lives; *"But the fruit of the Spirit is love, joy, peace, longsuffering, kindness, goodness, faithfulness, gentleness, self-control. Against such there is no law."* (Galatians 5:22 NKJV)*

Evil attitudes have to be done away with as a demonstration of true transformation. Thus, regardless of your religious affiliation – or the person that you dislike – we have to love one another and that love must be genuine and sacrificial.

Paul calls on us to be transformed; *"I beseech you therefore, brethren, by the mercies of God, that you present your bodies a living sacrifice, holy, acceptable to God, which is your reasonable service. And do not be conformed to this world, but be transformed by the renewing of your mind, that you may prove what is that good and acceptable and perfect will of God." (Romans 12:1-2 NKJV)**

This transformation is the beginning of a change that demonstrates our commitment to Him. In the process, God will show us what other things must be changed. We must realize that God will cause a total transformation to take place in us as we become more like His Son. From the way we think to the way we talk and act, everything must change so that we become more like Him, even how or how much we worship.

Does anyone truly believe that the Lord of the Sabbath will not honor the Sabbath during His reign? *"And He (Jesus) said to them, "The Son of Man is also Lord of the Sabbath." (Luke 6:5 NKJV)** Or can anyone deny that the festivals will not be celebrated during Christ's reign? *"And it shall come to pass that everyone who is left of all the nations which came against Jerusalem shall go up from year to year to worship the King, the LORD of hosts, and to keep the Feast of Tabernacles. And it shall be that whichever of the families of the earth do not come up to Jerusalem to worship the King, the LORD of hosts, on them there will be no rain. If the family of Egypt will not come up and enter in, they shall have no rain; they shall receive the plague with which the LORD strikes the nations who do not come up to keep the Feast of Tabernacles. This shall be the punishment* *of Egypt and the punishment of all the nations that do not come up to keep the Feast of Tabernacles." (Zechariah 14:16–19 NKJV)**

We may not be celebrating the feasts, and we can make up a lot of excuses for not celebrating the feasts. But since we will be observing them during Christ's millennial reign, according to the Word of God, why not start now?

We forget that God is the same yesterday, today, and forever. He does not change. What He celebrated in the past, He will celebrate in the future. These are Yahveh's feasts, holy assemblies that are to be perpetually celebrated. Yet most of the Christian churches ignore them.

With so many practices and beliefs and forms of worship, which of these, if any, will persist and continue in God's kingdom? I believe there are true believers in each religion that would be among God's select. If so, how would their differences be resolved? Our differences will be resolved by God, the one who will transform our bodies, *"Many nations shall come and say, 'Come, and let us go up to the mountain of the LORD, To the house of the God of Jacob; He will teach us His ways, And we shall walk in His paths.' For out of Zion the law shall go forth, And the word of the LORD from Jerusalem." (Micah 4:2 NKJV)** An ideal worshiper will be one that honors and obeys God for who He is, our great and almighty Creator.

With so many traditional Jews converting, the growth in Christian-Jewish (messianic) worship has greatly increased. This may have been God's plan in preserving traditional Judaism. Their continuance has permitted the resurgence of Jewish forms of worship, a sort of hybrid worship called Messianic worship.

This could be what God wants all faiths to do. Certainly a Shabbat service on Fridays, a Havdalah (end of the Sabbath) service on Saturdays, and a Son Rise or resurrection service on Sundays makes much more sense than the current religious designations and days of worship that most congregations have today.

Why are we worshiping on days that were not ordained by God? Is it for convenience? Have we forgotten our need to put God first? As servants of God, we should be doing that which would please Him and not what is convenient for us to do. We are failing to put God first.

Observing the feasts would be a good start. For one thing, there is much to learn that goes along with the feast that the church is missing out on. The feasts serve as a revelation of God's plan. They are the when, where, and how of God and His anointed Son Yahshua. The church should celebrate the feasts as God intended for His people to do.

This may be where we are headed. Certainly, the commanded observances and holy convocations, documented as observed by the ancient Israelites – along with the practice of sacrifices at the temple – are shown by the prophet Ezekiel to exist during Yahshua's thousand-year reign on Earth.

In both the books of Ezekiel and in Zechariah, temple worship with the priesthood and animal sacrifices exist in Israel during Christ's rule on earth. The description is clear: *"There was a chamber and its entrance by the gateposts of the gateway, where they washed the burnt offering. In the vestibule of the gateway were two tables on this side and two tables on that side, on which to slay the burnt offering, the sin offering, and the trespass offering. At the outer side* *of the vestibule, as one goes up to the entrance of the northern gateway, were two tables; and on the other side of the vestibule of the gateway were two tables. Four tables were on this side and four tables on that side, by the side of the gateway, eight tables on which they slaughtered the sacrifices. There were also four tables of hewn stone for the burnt offering, one cubit and a half long, one cubit and a half wide, and one cubit high; on these they laid the instruments with which they slaughtered the burnt offering and the sacrifice. Inside were hooks, a handbreadth wide, fastened all around; and the flesh of the sacrifices was on the tables." (Ezekiel 40:38–43 NKJV)**

In fact, the commanded observances and holy convocations are to be observed for all their generations. *"...it shall be a statute forever throughout your generations in all your dwellings." (Leviticus 23:14 NKJV)** This does not, however, preclude other Christ-established worships from taking place.

The continued sacrifices may be required as a reminder of the Jews' rejection of God's ultimate sacrifice, Jesus Christ, as a memorial.

In times past, God required holy convocations as a reminder so that the people would not forget where they had come from and what God had done.

Some Christians have a problem with this, as it is generally accepted that Christ was – and is – the final and full sacrifice. However, it is documented that during the first century, James (identified as of Jacob or Ya 'akov (בקעי) in the Jewish Talmud), as the high priest of the Essenes and other sects, continued during Yom Kippur to make atonement for his people. This was after Christ's crucifixion, despite recognizing the ultimate sacrifice that Christ had made.

James could have been continuing the sacrifices for those who had not yet come to repentance. We cannot be sure as to why James continued this practice, but the word does indicate that it will be conducted as well during the millenial reign of Christ. Perhaps, it is because it is commanded to be done "throughout your generations" and nowhere does it state that they are to stop.

We do not know exactly how worship will be or that it will be like anything any of us are doing today. But there is one thing we can be sure of: God will be honored. Make no mistake about it. God is in control. God wants us to be willing servants, servants that will honor and obey Him and do His will. He will teach us what He wants and how He wants it, as He has throughout the ages.

The period spoken of in Ezekiel and Zachariah occurs during the thousand-year reign of Christ, the end of which is marked by Satan being set loose and a rebellion. The sacrifices will be a point of contention during the later days of the reign. *"Then I saw an angel coming down from heaven, having the key to the bottomless pit and a great chain in his hand. He laid hold of the dragon, that serpent of old, who is the Devil and Satan, and bound him for a thousand years; and he cast him into the bottomless pit, and shut him up, and set a seal on him, so that he should deceive the nations no more till the thousand years were finished. But after these things he must be released for a little while."* (Revelation 20:1–3 NKJV)*

"And I saw thrones, and they sat on them, and judg-ment was committed to them. Then I saw the souls of those who had been beheaded for their witness to Jesus and for

the word of God, who had not worshiped the beast or his image, and had not received his mark on their foreheads or on their hands. And they lived and reigned with Christ for a thousand years. But the rest of the dead did not live again until the thousand years were finished. This is the first resurrection. Blessed and holy is he who has part in the first resurrection. Over such the second death has no power, but they shall be priests of God and of Christ, and shall reign with Him a thousand years." (Revelation 20:4–6 NKJV)*

"Now when the thousand years have expired, Satan will be released from his prison and will go out to deceive the nations which are in the four corners of the earth, Gog and Magog, to gather them together to battle, whose number is as the sand of the sea. They went up on the breadth of the earth and surrounded the camp of the saints and the beloved city. And fire came down from God out of heaven and devoured them. The devil, who deceived them, was cast into the lake of fire and brimstone where the beast and the false prophet are. And they will be tormented day and night forever and ever." (Revelation 20:7–10 NKJV)*

Chapter 14

1. The church is the body of _____, a body of people.

2. I do not know of a perfect _____, and I wonder, if Jesus Christ were to return today, where He would go to worship.

3. None of the customary practices that Jesus would have encountered in the Temple of His time are being practiced in _____ churches today.

4. It is obvious that God wants us _____ doing His work.

5. This is answered by the arrival of their redeemer Christ, who is believed to have actually been born during _____.

6. An ideal _____ will be one that honors and obeys God for who He is, our great and almighty Creator.

Answers: Christ, religion, Christian, busy, Tabernacles, worship

Chapter Fifteen

Your Purpose Must Fit into God's Plan

As stated in earlier chapters, God's purpose is to create a Kingdom of holy perfected subjects, the first of which is Christ Jesus. *"...to the general assembly and church of the firstborn who are registered in heaven, to God the Judge of all, to the spirits of just men made perfect..."* (Hebrews 12:23 NKJV)* *"He is the image of the invisible God, the firstborn over all creation. For by Him all things were created that are in heaven and that are on earth, visible and invisible, whether thrones or dominions or principalities or powers. All things were created through Him and for Him. And He is before all things, and in Him all things consist. And He is the head of the body, the church, who is the beginning, the firstborn from the dead, that in all things He may have the preeminence."* (Colossians 1:18 NKJV)* *And He said to them, "Go, tell that fox, 'Behold, I cast out demons and perform cures today and tomorrow, and the third day I shall be perfected.'"* (Luke 13:32 NKJV)*

Jesus the Son of God came to recruit souls for the Kingdom of God. He sent out His disciples with clear directives: *"And Jesus came and spoke to them, saying, "All authority has been given to Me in heaven and on earth. Go therefore and make disciples of all the nations, baptizing them in the name of the Father and of the Son and of the Holy Spirit, teaching them to observe all things that I have commanded you; and lo, I am with you always, even to the end of the age."* (Matthew 27:16–20 NKJV)*

As His followers we are commanded likewise to make disciples of all nations. We have, therefore, the task of becoming like Him as followers and of duplicating ourselves by making followers of others. This forms our core purpose. We are to follow the directives written in the gospel accounts of Jesus.

We may take this task lightly, but the fact is that there is much to gain if we do as Christ commands and much to lose if we do not. Is there a better offer than to add to God's kingdom? Is there a more valuable reward or a better option? The Bible states that our life is like a vapor, here today and gone tomorrow. Only the eternal has any real value. *"Come now, you who say, 'Today or tomorrow we will go to such and such a city, spend a year there, buy and sell, and make a profit;' whereas you do not know what will happen tomorrow. For what is your life? It is even a vapor that appears for a little time and then vanishes away. Instead you ought to say, 'If the Lord wills, we shall live and do this or that.' But now you boast in your arrogance. All such boasting is evil."* (James 4:13–16 NKJV)*

Most people spend all of their money and efforts on projects that have no eternal reward. They build their empires ignoring God. But ignore God, and He will ignore you. Can someone who does not give God one's most prized possession, his or her life, expect to get God's most prized reward?

God's offer is better than any investment anyone could make, and it is eternal. God offers life and not just life as we know it but life incorruptible, transformed into the ideal, the same as the resurrected body of Christ Jesus.

I do not believe that Christ was crucified at the age of thirty-three years by pure chance. The age of thirty-three is a peak age for the human body. If we were to be transformed into the ideal, peak age would be the optimum age to be transformed into. Regardless of the age of death, a person being brought back would be best brought back at peak age and in perfect health. The age of thirty-three is a perfect option.

This applies to everyone, even to the children that did not have a chance at life or died before responsibility was imposed on them. To the older ones, their lives and their decisions, for or against God and His anointed, will determine their fate.

We are called to be perfect, to be like Christ. This is what God wants of us. Paul advised Jesus' followers to be transformed, to be holy. *"I beseech you therefore, brethren, by the mercies of God, that you present your bodies a living sacrifice, holy, acceptable to God, which is your reasonable service. And do not be conformed to this world, but be transformed by the renewing of your mind, that you may prove what is that good and acceptable and perfect will of God." (Romans 12:1–2 NKJV)**

The greatest tools for transformation are the application of God's word and prayer. Learning by imitating requires putting into practice that which one has learned. With practice, the actions become spontaneous reactions that form a part of the person's being. These changes are identified as fruits of the spirit because it is the Spirit which guides you during the transformation process. *"But the fruit of the Spirit is love, joy, peace, longsuffering, kindness, goodness, faithfulness, gentleness, self-control." (Galatians 5:22–23 NKJV)** All are qualities or fruits that we must exhibit.

Jesus taught that we are to produce such fruit and that those who do not will be cut away. *"I am the true vine, and My Father is the vinedresser. Every branch in Me that does not bear fruit He takes away; and every branch that bears fruit He prunes, that it may bear more fruit." (John 15:1–2 NKJV)** God, through our trials and tribulations, makes our lives more fruitful.

This fruit bearing comes by abiding in Christ through prayer and application of God's Word. *"Abide in Me, and I in you. As the branch cannot bear fruit of itself, unless it abides in the vine, neither can you, unless you abide in Me. I am the vine, you are the branches. He who abides in Me, and I in him, bears much fruit; for without Me you can do nothing. If anyone does not abide in Me, he is cast out as a branch and is withered; and they gather them and throw them into the fire, and they are burned. If you abide in Me, and My words abide in you, you will ask what you desire, and it shall be done for you. By this My Father is glorified, that you bear much fruit; so you will be My disciples." (John 15:4–8 NKJV)**

The "what-would-Jesus-do movement" is an attempt to help individuals in their life decisions so as to become more like Jesus. This is fine. But it only scratches the surface when it comes to the holiness-transformation requirement spoken of by Paul in Romans 12:1 and 2.

We will not be truly holy until our bodies are glorified at the return of Christ. While we are still in this earthly body, we are to honor Christ by being like Him in our choices, desires, and responses. We must not conform to the ways, attitudes, or values that the worldly, materialistic, and self-indulging person gives in to.

A powerful tool in this respect is prayer. Having intimate personal communion with God in prayer is a powerfully transforming process. This has been the turning point in many great evangelists and followers of Christ and something that many have failed to comprehend. There is a transformation and empowering that occurs when one spends time alone with God. Persistence and perseverance seems to be a major catalyst in this process which is why the Bible tells us to pray without ceasing. *"Rejoice always, pray without ceasing, in everything give thanks; for this is the will of God in Christ Jesus for you."* (1 Thessalonians 5:16–18 NKJV)*

Our family was Catholic up to my eleventh birthday. Afterwards, we attended a Methodist church until my fourteenth birthday when my family began attending a Pentecostal church which I also occasionally attended.

A practice in the Pentecostal church which caused a major change in my mother's prayer life was the all-night prayer vigils that they had. People would be on their knees or walking around praying out loud. It was quite a moving experience. Many had what is called as the gift of the Holy Spirit which gave them a strong desire and the endurance to take part in the all night event. Participating in the vigils brought my mother to a higher level of holiness which I had not seen in her before. She seemed wiser and sharper, and her devotion to God more profound. It was with these experiences that my mother could spend hours on her knees praying as she did many nights.

I can recall when my little brother was about three years old. He had gotten a viral infection of his eyes, and despite my mother's prayers, he continued to worsen. I remember how one day my mother came home in tears because the doctor had told her that my brother could lose his vision. The sclera, or white of his eyes, were so swollen that the dark irises were buried in the white sclera. I can recall my mother laying him down on her bed and praying over him, pleading with God to spare his eyes. She prayed all through the night without ever going to sleep. In the morning, she got up and went to work as she always did. Later that morning, my brother awoke, his eyes appearing completely normal. My mother's perseverance paid off.

This may sound way out for some, but what we forget is that such experiences mold us into the person God wants us to be. We oftentimes get tired of asking God to intervene for us or to assist us with some problem, not knowing that provisions for the answer were made long before we asked. Sometimes, God does not answer the way we would like Him to answer because we do not see the whole picture, and He does. I have seen many come to Christ through the death of a loved one. I have seen miraculously healed individuals become lost and die in their sins. Sometimes, a denial is a better answer. Yet, we should be asking with perseverance since the experience may be the objective of His answer.

A good example of this is the story of Jacob wrestling with the Angel of God for a blessing. *"Then Jacob was left alone; and a Man wrestled with him until the breaking of day. Now when He saw that He did not prevail against him, He touched the socket of his hip; and the socket of Jacob's hip was out of joint as He wrestled with him. And He said, 'Let Me go, for the day breaks.' But he said, 'I will not let You go unless You bless me!' So He said to him, 'What is your name?' He said, 'Jacob.' And He said, 'Your name shall no longer be called Jacob, but Israel; for you have struggled with God and with men, and have prevailed.' Then Jacob asked, saying, "Tell me Your name, I pray." And He said, 'Why is it that you ask about My name?' And He blessed him there. So Jacob called the name of the place Peniel: 'For I*

*have seen God face to face, and my life is preserved.'"
(Genesis 32:24–30 NKJV)**

Despite his pain and fatigue, Jacob would not let the angel go. Would we be as persistent, or would we give up long before this? God wants us to be persistent, tenacious, and unswerving towards the things of God and those things which are rightfully for our blessing. This forms part of our transformation as it did for Jacob who from henceforth became "Israel," which can be interpreted as "persevering with God."

Each person needs to understand God's plan for himself while working to grow God's plan for mankind. Revealing God's plan is number one. Sharing and caring and building up the body of believers to achieve greater growth is the method.

Unfortunately all too often, the greatest obstacle to the growth of Christianity is the Christians themselves, due to their poor examples. They get dragged down by the very same things that those out of the church get entangled with. I can still remember reading the biography of Mahatma Ghandi, wherein he makes the statement, "I would be a Christian if not for Christians." This is a terrible indictment of those who supposedly serve the living God.

Corruption, divorce, and infidelity are devastating the Christian faith. About half of Christian marriages end up in divorce. It appears many Christians do not practice the very things that they preach. They are more interested in pleasing their desires than on pleasing God.

Christianity has become so commercialized that the great majority of leaders are looking at the bottom line —

the dollar — instead of preserving their relationship with God.

Many have become like the merchants on the temple steps, delving in areas they know they should not be, conducting business in a manner that dishonors God. To them Christ says, ".... "It is written, 'My house shall be called a house of prayer,' but you have made it a 'den of thieves." (Matthew 21:13 NKJV)* They defile God's temple, which today is the body of Christ.

The poor spouse is left with putting up with the humiliation or parting ways. In both instances it is a devastation of life. The families, particularly the children, the followers, and associates, are all affected. The worse thing of all is the victory gained by God's enemy and the rejection of God that ensues because of the poor examples.

Every follower should have a regular and continuous routine, wherein their tank is filled up again. Whether it is a particular day or week of continous fasting and prayer or whatever it is that a person can fit into their schedule, they need to prostrate themselves before God and let Him fill them up again.

An individual should work at nourishing their spirit regularly in addition to their routine participation in worshiping and fellowship with others. One has to purpose in their heart not to be a stumbling block to anyone but to serve as an example to others and to be able to say as Paul said, "Imitate me as I imitate Christ".

For those who come across such poor examples, do not let it be a barrier to you establishing a relationship with the God of the universe. Someday you will stand before Him and have to give account for your rejection. You will not be able to point to another person since your example is Christ.

We must follow the advice given to us by Paul, *"For I say, through the grace given to me, to everyone who is among you, not to think of himself more highly than he ought to think, but to think soberly, as God has dealt to each one a measure of faith. For as we have many members in one body, but all the members do not have the same function, so we, being many, are one body in Christ, and individually members of one another. Having then gifts differing according to the grace that is given to us, let us use them: if prophecy, let us prophesy in proportion to our faith; or ministry, let us use it in our ministering; he who teaches, in teaching; he who exhorts, in exhortation; he who gives, with liberality; he who leads, with diligence; he who shows mercy, with cheerfulness. Let love be without hypocrisy. Abhor what is evil. Cling to what is good. Be kindly affectionate to one another with brotherly love, in honor giving preference to one another; not lagging in diligence, fervent in spirit, serving the Lord; rejoicing in hope, patient in tribulation, continuing steadfastly in prayer; distributing to the needs of the saints, given to hospitality. Bless those who persecute you; bless and do not curse. Rejoice with those who rejoice, and weep with those who weep. Be of the same mind toward one another. Do not set your mind on high things, but associate with the humble. Do not be wise in your own opinion. Repay no one evil for evil. Have regard for good things in the sight of all men. If it is possible, as much as depends on you, live peaceably with all men."(Romans 12:3-18 NKJV)**

Christians must shed their past and not let them-selves become contaminated with the corruptive forces that are in this world. Christ explained, *"But those things which proceed out of the mouth come from the heart, and they* *defile a man. For out of the heart proceed evil thoughts, murders, adulteries, fornications, thefts, false witness, and blasphemies. These are the things which defile a man, . . ." (Matthew 15:18-20 NKJV)**

The ancient Hebrews used the word heart (lev or לב) as the seat of all thoughts, the authority of the brain and all emotions. In the great commandment, *"You shall love the LORD your God with all your heart, with all your soul, and with all your strength." (Deuteronomy 6:5 NKJV)** "Heart" implies, with all your thoughts and emotions, your mind is to be consumed with thoughts of the Almighty. The word "soul" implies life or living body or organs. The moving back and forth of the Jews at the Wailing Wall while praying is a demostration of worshiping God with their "soul," i.e. their body. The word "strength" is the measure that God has given you or all that you own i.e. your money.

When Jesus spoke from the heart, He was speaking from the perspective of the seat of the mind. We must, therefore, seek to have a pure heart, to despise those things that God does not approve of. If we are to be perfected — if we are to reveal the divinity of Christ in us — than we must have a heart like Christ.

In his book <u>Mysteries of the Kingdom Revealed</u>, the author Luis Caquias points out that it is what enters a person that is expressed by the mouth or heart that corrupts a person — in modern day parlance "junk in, junk out."

What enters through the eyes and ears that corrupt is what taints your heart. Just as what edifies can enter the heart through the eyes and ears, so what corrupts enters through the eyes and ears. For this reason, a person wanting to please God protects his heart from corruption by keeping from corruptive visual and audible messages.

We must understand that God's purpose for us is that we become like His son. We are to become as Christ in word, thought, and actions. It is not just our body that must be transformed but also our mind. God's spirit will guide us, but we have the option to accept or reject what is presented to us. We must choose those things that edify our Spirit and reject all that corrupts. We must desire holiness. If we seek God, to have a closer walk with Him, there is no exception.

Chapter 15

1. God's purpose is to create a kingdom of holy perfected subjects, the first of which is _____.

2. We have, therefore, the task of _____ like Him as followers and of duplicating ourselves by making followers of others.

3. The Bible says that our life is like a _____.

4. Most people spend all of their money and efforts on projects that have no eternal _____.

5. Can someone who does not give God one's most _____ possession, his or her life, expect to get God's most prized reward?

6. God wants us to be _____, tenacious, and unswerving towards the things of God and those things which are rightfully for our blessing.

Answers: Christ Jesus, becoming, vapor, reward, prized, persistent

Chapter Sixteen

The Conflicts

One of the obstacles encountered when confronted with the concept of God during modern times is how the various findings in nature and science fit into the concept of a creator God.

Considering the age of the earth as supposedly established by science and the fossil record and all of the evolutionary concepts, how can someone accept the concept of a creator God? This was for me the greatest of obstacles while growing up. As I gained more knowledge, I realized that life was a lot more complex than I imagined it to be. After pondering about all of the complexities in life, I concluded that only by deliberate design could life have come about.

The Bible in the book of Job describes an animal that could be a dinosaur though science claims they were to have vanished by the time man came into existence. In the book of Job one finds: *"Look now at the behemoth, which I made along with you; He eats grass like an ox. See now, his strength is in his hips, and his power is in his stomach muscles. He moves his tail like a cedar; the sinews of his thighs are tightly knit. His bones are like beams of bronze, His ribs like bars of iron. He is the first of the ways of God; Only He who made him can bring near His sword. Surely the mountains yield food for him, and all the beasts of the field play there. He lies under the lotus trees, in a covert of reeds and marsh. The lotus trees cover him with their shade; the willows by the brook surround him. Indeed the river may* rage, yet he is not disturbed; He is confident, though the Jordan gushes into his mouth, though he takes it in his eyes, or one pierces his nose with a snare." (Job 40:15–24 NKJV)*

This describes an animal with a cedar tree-like tail and a strong front torso, large with strong thighs and a prominent chest. Certainly, this could not be an elephant, a mammoth, a hippopotamus, or a rhinoceros. You cannot see the ribs on a hippopotamus, and its tail is like that of a pig as is the rhinoceros' tail.

The Jordon River is 90 to 100 feet wide. The expression "the river may rage, yet he is not disturbed; He is confident, though the Jordan gushes into his mouth," and that it lies under shade trees and requires mountains of food implies that this must have been a truly large animal like a dinosaur and not like any animal we know of today. It also claims that this creature was a first or earlier creation of God which falls in line with the fossil record.

There is also another creature in the Bible which is called a leviathan, a sea creature which apparently was known of during Job's time. In Psalms and Job, the power of the leviathan is alluded to. "Can you draw out Leviathan with a hook, or snare his tongue with a line which you lower? Can you put a reed through his nose, or pierce his jaw with a hook? Will he make many supplications to you? Will he speak softly to you? Will he make a covenant with you? Will you take him as a servant forever? Will you play with him as with a bird, or will you leash him for your maidens? Will your companions make a banquet of him? Will they apportion him among the merchants? Can you fill his skin with harpoons, or his head with fishing spears? Lay your hand on him; Remember the battle; Never do it again! Indeed, any hope of overcoming him is false; shall one not be overwhelmed at the sight of him? No one is so fierce that he would dare stir him up. Who then is able to stand against Me?" (Job 41:1–10 NKJV)*

This sea creature is also described in the book of Psalms. *"O LORD, how manifold are Your works! In wisdom You have made them all. The earth is full of Your possessions. This great and wide sea, in which are innumerable teeming things, Living things both small and great. There the ships sail about. There is that Leviathan which You have made to play there."* (Psalms 106:24–26 NKJV)*

This creature, the leviathan, has become synonymous with sea serpent or dragon and, according to the description, was quite large and fierce unlike any known living creature of today.

One can believe that such creatures did not exist, that they were simply fabrications of the writer's imagination, but such assumptions are less credible then that these creatures were known, real, and eye-witnessed, as evidenced by their inclusion in these writings. The authors are using their description to demonstrate the greater power of the creator God; thus, obviously, the authors had first-hand knowledge of these creatures and include them because they were real to them.

God is creator of all things. From the innumerable types of living creatures and vast number of planetary bodies, it is readily apparent that God loves to create. Could there be other planets or universes with similar life forms created for God's purpose? Of course, there could be. But would it make any difference? Would it take anything away from God's purpose? It is God's prerogative. He can do what He wants when He wants. He does not need anyone's permission. He creates all types of life and chooses whom He wills to fulfill His plan.

From the number of species and tremendous size of the universe, one thing that we can say is that God likes to do things in big ways. It would not surprise me to learn that God had similar creations elsewhere. Just as we like having homes in different cities, God may very well like having kingdoms in different galaxies for His glory.

As stated in prior chapters, creation by natural selection (what we used to know as evolution) is unproven, and there is more evidence against it than there is for it. It is a destructive doctrine since its premise is that we came about spontaneously – God is not needed. Diversity among the species is now called evolution, a deviant scheme to make evolution acceptable. Without a doubt, this is a demonic scheme and an attack on the creator God.

To say that God used natural selection to bring about life is to consider God as not being supernatural. God would be bound by the same laws of nature as we are – He would not be God.

God is not bound by the Laws of nature; He established the laws of nature. He makes them do what ever He wants. He is a supernatural God. He is not a God who has to mind the limits of physical laws.

Neither time nor space can restrict Him. He is omniscient, omnipresent, and omnipotent. He controls time and space. All energy is at His command. Nothing that is would be without Him. His power holds no limit. He is soveriegn over all.

If creation by natural selection or evolution were the way life forms came into existence, we would all be asexual beings. We would be reproducing by a method like budding – asexual reproduction – rather than by such a complicated system as sexual reproduction. The millions of life forms that reproduce by sexual reproduction attest to the impossibility of creation by natural selection or evolution.

Sexual reproduction requires that two highly complicated organisms evolve simultaneously, thus doubling the complexities required of natural selection. This is complicated a billion fold by the many millions of organisms having similar requirements.

Any principled molecular geneticist can attest to the prerequisite knowledge and complexity involved in undertaking the task of gene transfer for a single variant. The task of creating a completely different species or even a single cell organism from simple organic chemicals is immensly more difficult if not impossible. Unfortunately, gene transfer is now deliberately being labeled as evolution, and the variant is now considered a new species, adding greater confusion to the evolution creation argument.

Spontaneity in nature always follows the path of least resistance, that is, the easiest way out – law of maximized entropy – and not the path of maximized complexity.

Humans are relational beings, made in the image of God who is Himself a relational being. The first union of a man and a woman is a covenant act sealed with blood. This is evidence of God's creation and participation in the establishment of marriage between a man and a woman. The spilling of blood is God's principal method of sealing a commitment.

There is not a conflict with divine creation and man's findings in those who accept the existence of an all powerful, supernatural God. They accept and believe divine creation by faith, *"...faith is the substance of things hoped for, the evidence of things not seen."* (Hebrews 11:1 NKJV)*... *"But without faith it is impossible to please Him, for he who comes to God must believe that He is, and that He is a rewarder of those who diligently seek Him."* (Hebrews 11:2 NKJV)*

Unbelievers are driven by their attempt to make sense of this world without a supernatural creator God. They begin with the false premise that there is no supernatural God and that we came about by natural means. Nothing can change their minds since they believe that their premise is correct despite violating the very laws all other physical laws are based on. They have developed their own faith that is backed up by nothing but presumption. This is true perversion and foolishness. They ignore the findings and continue to seek a truth that does not exist at times denying even that Jesus ever existed, a totally illogical and nonsense assumption.

The unbelievers have many recruits. For many have been deceived and bought the lie, refusing to believe the impossibility of creation by natural selection or that they would be held accountable to an all knowing and powerful God.

They argue the scientific method yet deny the very basis of science — the strict adherence to the tried and tested laws by which all science is measured. Creation by natural selection fails by being non-compliant to the second law of thermodynamics. Thus, based on science and not on opinion, creation by natural selection is impossible.

Individuals controlling the media and the educational institutions push the creation by natural selection evolution doctrine while suppressing divine creation. Their position of influence puts them in the same position as are church leaders which are held to a stricter standard. God has a very special place reserved for these folks in the lake of fire.

Fathoming God from a mere human perspective is an impossible task. The Bible tells us that God is not in the universe but that the universe is in God; " 'Can anyone hide himself in secret places, So I shall not see him?' says the LORD; 'Do I not fill heaven and earth?' says the LORD." (Jeremiah 23:24 NKJV)*

Isaiah declares that God measures the entire universe with a span, the distance between the tip of the thumb and the pinky of one hand; "Who has measured the waters in the hollow of His hand, Measured heaven with a span And calculated the dust of the earth in a measure? Weighed the mountains in scales And the hills in a balance?" (Isaiah 40:12 NKJV)*

Can anyone with knowledge of the immensity of the universe conceptualize God from the prospective of all things in the universe being in Him? Can anyone conceptualize God measuring the universe with His hand? It is so much beyond our comprehension that it would be foolish for anyone to try. Can we measure God? Are we so foolish as to try? There are some things that one must just simply accept.

It has not been very long ago since the discovery that there are innumerable galaxies. We have learned through the use of our telescope technology like the Hubble telescope that throughout the universe there are over a hundred billion galaxies which contain over a hundred billion stars like our sun. The shear size and number of these celestial bodies is so incredible that it is impossible to comprehend.

There is only one book which accurately documents and predates the actual findings and discoveries of the celestial bodies by thousands of years and that book is the Bible. While Hindu tradition taught that the earth was resting on the backs of several huge elephants and Greek mythology claimed that the god Atlas was holding the earth on his shoulders, the Bible proclaimed, " *God hangeth the earth on nothing,*" "*He stretches out the north over empty space; He hangs the earth on nothing.*" *(Job 26:7 NKJV)**

As stated elsewhere, while people believed the world was flat, God's word revealed it to be round nearly three thousand years before it was discovered. "*It is He who sits above the circle of the earth...,*" *(Isaiah 40:22 NKJV)**

The book of Job also describes a circle in its description of the heavens; "*Thick clouds cover Him, so that He cannot see, And He walks above the circle of heaven.*" *(Job 22:14 NKJV)** Proverbs 8 also describes earth as a circle; "*When He prepared the heavens, I was there, "When He drew a circle on the face of the deep,*" *(Proverbs 8:27 NKJV)**

Until modern times, the bottom of the oceans were believed to be sandy plains while the Bible, thousands of years before, revealed the ocean bottom to contain mountains and valleys and large crevices. "*The waters surrounded me, even to my soul; The deep closed around me; Weeds were wrapped around my head. I went down to the moorings of the mountains; The earth with its bars closed behind me forever; Yet You have brought up my life from the pit, O LORD, my God.*" *(Jonah 2:5-6 NKJV)** "*Then* the channels of the sea were seen, The foundations of the world were uncovered...." (Psalm 18:15 NKJV)*

Over three thousands years ago, Psalms revealed that there were paths or currents, rivers of water, that course through our oceans that were unknown until their discovery in the 1800's by Matthew Maury—the father of Modern Navigation. *"The birds of the air, And the fish of the sea that pass through the paths of the seas."(Psalm 8:8 NKJV)*

While all other religious books created many superstitious tales to explain the weather and rain, the Bible accurately taught that the weather follows specific rules and cycles. *"While the earth remains, Seedtime and harvest, Cold and heat, winter and summer, And day and night Shall not cease." (Genesis 8:22 NKJV)** The Bible revealed without science what man later was to learn through science, *"When He made a law for the rain, And a path for the thunderbolt," (Job 28:26 NKJV)** He who builds His layers in the sky, And has founded His strata in the earth; Who calls for the waters of the sea, And pours them out on the face of the earth— The LORD (Yahveh) is His name." (Amos 9:6 NKJV)**

The book of Job reveals some amazing astronomical facts which modern science has only recently been able to discover; *"Can you bind the cluster of the Pleiades, Or loose the belt of Orion? Can you bring out Mazzaroth in its season? Or can you guide the Great Bear with its cubs?" (Job 38:31-32 NKJV)**

Modern observation methods have revealed that the Pleiades is a cluster of some 500 stars that are moving in the same direction bound by forces to each other. In Job, God takes credit for their binding and asks Job if he can accomplish such a feat.

The belt of Orion consist as a pattern of stars in the constellation Orion which is consistantly seen together as three bright stars. God ask Job, "Are you able to loosen the belt of Orion?" The implication here is that God could if He so desired because He put them there.

Mazzaroth are constellations that are seen in the sky differing with the seasons. God takes credit for these as well as He does for the Great Bear (Ursa Major) with its cubs (Ursa Minor). The Big Dipper is a part of the Great Bear which points to the North Star. The North Star is part of the Little Dipper seen at the end of its handle. God takes credit for creating and guiding these constellations.

While many feel that discoveries in science conflict with findings in scripture, the exact opposite is true. The Bible has revealed many things before they were known. Science discovered mechanisms and rules in nature that were well-established in the Bible before their discovery. What fool would challenge a God with the evidence that there is in the scriptures and all around us? Only a fool would say there is no God!

There is no conflict with science, only unbelief. People refuse to believe that there could be a supernatural God who is responsible for all creation. Many cling to wanting to see Him first in order to believe, but God chooses not to show Himself, relying instead on the evidence that He has provided to demonstrate Himself to us.

God hates pride and arrogance. *"To fear the LORD is to hate evil; I hate pride and arrogance, evil behavior and perverse speech."* (Proverbs 8:13 NKJV)* At the root of all rejection of God is a prideful heart; *"In his pride the wicked does not seek him; in all his thoughts there is no room for*

God." (Psalm 10:4 NKJV)* If God were to present Himself, He would be giving in to a prideful wicked heart which He hates and wants no part of.

Some people argue that they are not wicked because they do not believe in God. They do not have any malice against the concept of a creator God but simply do not believe that He exists.

This would be true if God did not exist, but if He does, the mere rejection is a malicious act. The denial of your creator, who created a place for you, who gave you life and an eternal paradise reward is outright malicious. It is more than just a mere lack of appreciation since He is not your equal; He is "God."

Your rejection not only affects you but also affects your children and their descendents. *"My people are destroyed for lack of knowledge. Because you have rejected knowledge, I also will reject you from being priest for Me; because you have forgotten the law of your God, I also will forget your children." (Hosea 4:6 NKJV)* *"...For I, the LORD your God, am a jealous God, visiting the iniquity of the fathers upon the children to the third and fourth generations of those who hate Me," (Exodus 20:5 NKJV)* Those who believe and serve God, He makes His priest.

Individuals who worship false gods, who continue despite the evidence of them being false gods, are in the same situation as any atheist who rejects the creator God. Imagine if God would bless an individual for bringing Him his tithes, how much more blessings He would give for giving of himself. *"Bring all the tithes into the storehouse, That there may be food in My house, And try Me now in this," says the LORD of hosts, "If I will not open for you the windows of heaven And pour out for you such blessing That there will not be room enough to receive it."*

God wants humble, caring, confiding, and obedient servants. He does not care for those who reject Him. He loves those that love Him. *"I love those who love me, and those who seek me find me." (Proverbs 8:17 NKJV)** He has provided proof of His creation. You have read the evidence, so the rest is up to you!

Chapter 16

1. The Bible in the book of Job describes an animal that could be a _____ though science claims they were to have vanished by the time man came into existence.

2. Certainly, this could not be an elephant, a mammoth, a _____, or a rhinoceros.

3. It claims that a _____ river would not disturb this animal even if it were to go into his mouth or eyes.

4. One can believe that such creatures did not exist, that they were simply _____ of the writer's imagination, but such assumptions are less credible then that these creatures were real, known, and eye-witnessed as evidence by their inclusion in these writings.

5. From the innumerable types of living creatures and innumerable planetary bodies, it is readily apparent that God _____ to create.

6. He creates all types of life and _____ whom He wills to fulfill His plan.

Answers: dinosaur, hippopotamus, raging, fabrications, loves, chooses

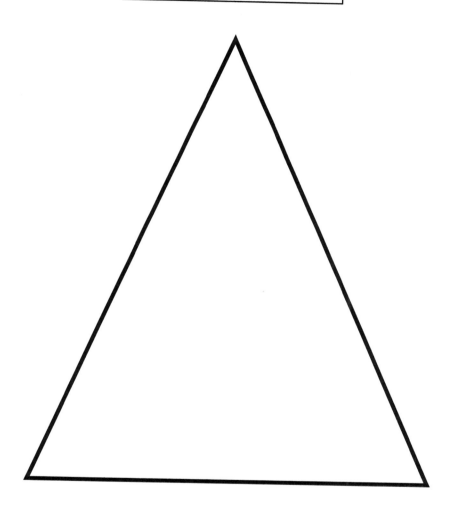

GOD'S DISTANCE

MAN'S DISTANCE

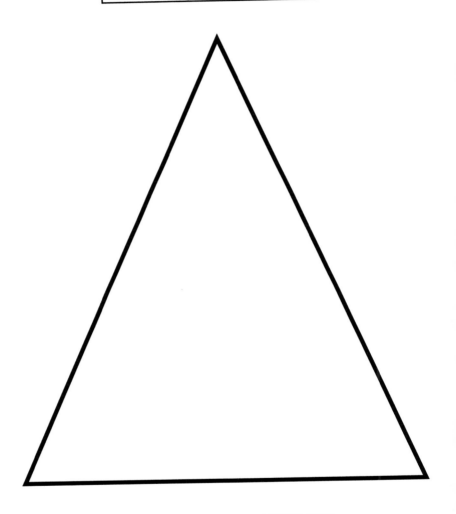

GOD'S TIME

MAN'S TIME

Chapter Seventeen

The Creation

In the book of Genesis, we learn that God made man. There are two separate accounts. In Genesis 1, we read that on the sixth day God made man. *Then God said, "'Let Us make man in Our image, according to Our likeness; let them have dominion over the fish of the sea, over the birds of the air, and over the cattle, over all the earth and over every creeping thing that creeps on the earth.' So God created man in His own image; in the image of God He created him; male and female He created them. Then God blessed them, and God said to them, 'Be fruitful and multiply; fill the earth and subdue it; have dominion over the fish of the sea, over the birds of the air, and over every living thing that moves on the earth.'" (Genesis 1:26–28 NKJV)**

In Genesis 2, we read: *"And the LORD God formed man of the dust of the ground, and breathed into his nostrils the breath of life; and man became a living being. The LORD God planted a garden eastward in Eden, and there He put the man whom He had formed." (Genesis 2:7–8 NKJV)**

God blessed Adam with a spouse called Eve, formed from his rib. *"And the LORD God caused a deep sleep to fall on Adam, and he slept; and He took one of his ribs, and closed up the flesh in its place. Then the rib which the LORD God had taken from man He made into a woman, and He brought her to the man." (Genesis 2:21–22 NKJV)**

As to whether Genesis 1 and 2 refers to the same person or to different persons, it is generally accepted that it is referring to the same event with more details in the second chapter. In other areas of the Bible, Adam is identified as the first man, *"And so it is written, 'The first man Adam became a living being.' The last Adam became a life-giving spirit."* (1 Corinthians 15:45 NKJV)* None of these interpretations changes God's plan or His relationship with man.

Certain faiths consider the Genesis account a myth, but such assessment denies the supernatural nature of God. Genesis is an allegory. An allegory is a description of one thing with the image of another. It is not untrue. A myth is fictitious. The Bible was written so that everyone could understand it. Parables used by Jesus in His teachings were frequently allegorical. That Genesis should be written in the same manner is not out of the ordinary.

Some say that the account in Genesis 1 is evidence that there were other people on Earth before Adam. Were there others placed outside the Garden of Eden and a selected individual placed in the Garden of Eden from whom we descended through Noah's children? Was Adam called "first man" because he was the first homo sapien, or was he called the "first man" because he was the first selected by God for His great and glorious plan?

Adam was given a soul, as it states that God "breathed into his nostrils the breath of life; and man became a living being." Were the others without a soul? Can those be the other hominids that have been found, or are they from a pre-Adam era?

The concept of Genesis 1 being pre–Adam is an attempt by some to fit the fossil record and the scientific findings of today into the Genesis account. Those opposed argue that there was no death prior to Adam's sin so that there could not have existed disease and death prior to Adam as is seen in the fossil record.

The belief by the pre-Adam believers, The Gap theorist, is that there were other men with the fallen angels and Lucifer on the pre-Adam earth. God destroyed them with earthquakes, volcanoes, and a great flood for their defiance and evil. The earth was left empty and void and covered by crystalline ash, creating darkness that did not permit the sun to penetrate the surface of the earth, *"The likeness of the firmament above the heads of the living creatures was like the color of an awesome crystal, stretched out over their heads." (Ezekiel 1:22 NKJV)**

Volcanic ash could very well cover the earth and not let the sun rays penetrate the surface, causing everything to die and with the flood covering the mountains leaving the earth without form, and void, and in darkness as described in Genesis 1:2. The Adamic age is said to have begun with the creation of Adam in which God put forth His plan to create perfect beings.

The argument that there could not be death prior to Adam may not be applicable to those prior to Adam. These prior individuals could have been discounted by God for the same reason that they were destroyed. Disobedience and unbelief appears to be a cause for God blotting out an individual or individuals from His word as He will do to those who do not believe and defy Him in the current era.

An example of this is the story of Abraham and Isaac. While the first born son of Abraham was actually Ishmael, God discounted Ishmael because he was the child of disobedience and unbelief. God instead asked Abraham to sacrifice Isaac whom He called Abraham's only son when in fact Isaac was not Abraham's only son; *"Now Sarai, Abram's wife, had borne him no children. And she had an Egyptian* maidservant whose name was Hagar. So Sarai said to Abram, 'See now, the LORD has restrained me from bearing children. Please, go in to my maid; perhaps I shall obtain children by her.' And Abram heeded the voice of Sarai. Then Sarai, Abram's wife, took Hagar her maid, the Egyptian, and gave her to her husband Abram to be his wife, after Abram had dwelt ten years in the land of Canaan. So he went in to Hagar, and she conceived...." (Genesis 16:1-4 NKJV)*" "So Hagar bore Abram a son; and Abram named his son, whom Hagar bore, Ishmael." (Genesis 16:15 NKJV)*

Abraham then fell on his face, laughed, and said in his heart, "Shall a child be born to a man who is one hundred years old? And shall Sarah, who is ninety years old, bear a child?" And Abraham said to God, "Oh, that Ishmael might live before You!" Then God said: "No, Sarah your wife shall bear you a son, and you shall call his name Isaac; I will establish My covenant with him for an everlasting covenant, and with his descendants after him. And as for Ishmael, I have heard you. Behold, I have blessed him, and will make him fruitful, and will multiply him exceedingly. He shall beget twelve princes, and I will make him a great nation. But My covenant I will establish with Isaac, whom Sarah shall bear to you at this set time next year." Then He finished talking with him, and God went up from Abraham. So Abraham took Ishmael his son, all who were born in his house and all who were bought with his money, every male among the men of Abraham's house, and circumcised the flesh of their foreskins that very same day, as God had said to him. Abraham was ninety-nine years old when he was circumcised in the flesh of his foreskin. And Ishmael his son was thirteen years old when he was circumcised in the flesh of his foreskin. That very same day Abraham was circumcised, and his son Ishmael; and all the men of his house, born in the house or bought with money from a foreigner, were circumcised with him." (Genesis 17:17-27 NKJV)*

"And He said, 'I will certainly return to you according to the time of life, and behold, Sarah your wife shall have a son.' (Sarah was listening in the tent door which was behind him.) Now Abraham and Sarah were old, well advanced in age; and Sarah had passed the age of childbearing. Therefore Sarah laughed within herself, saying, 'After I have grown old, shall I have pleasure, my lord being old also?' And the LORD said to Abraham, 'Why did Sarah laugh, saying, "Shall I surely bear a child, since I am old?" Is anything too hard for the LORD? At the appointed time I will return to you, according to the time of life, and Sarah shall have a son.' But Sarah denied it, saying, 'I did not laugh,' for she was afraid. And He said, 'No, but you did laugh!' (Genesis 18:10-15 NKJV)* And the LORD visited Sarah as He had said, and the LORD did for Sarah as He had spoken. For Sarah conceived and bore Abraham a son in his old age, at the set time of which God had spoken to him. And Abraham called the name of his son who was born to him—whom Sarah bore to him—Isaac. Then Abraham circumcised his son Isaac when he was eight days old, as God had commanded him." (Genesis 21:1-4 NKJV)* "Now it came to pass after these things that God tested Abraham, and said to him, 'Abraham!'And he said, 'Here I am.' Then He said, 'Take now your son, your only son Isaac, whom you love, and go to the land of Moriah, and offer him there as a burnt offering on one of the mountains of which I shall tell you.'" (Genesis 22:1-2 NKJV)*

The point to this is that if God discounted Ishmael because of Abraham's and Sarah's disorbedience then God could have discounted any people who may have been around prior to Adam for the same reason.

I am not endorsing any of the Genesis explanations. Either one of these is plausible; only God truly knows. God gave us as much as He felt was necessary in His word. After all, He is God. Paul advised that we should avoid disputes that generate strife, *"But avoid foolish and ignorant disputes, knowing that they generate strife." (2 Timothy 2:23 NKJV)**

Individuals who adhere to the strict literal interpretation of the Bible create stumbling blocks for any intellectual attempting to make sense out of the biblical account. God reigns superior; He does what He does any way that He wants to. We are but to accept it and not try to second guess Him. This is what God told Job when Job questioned Him as to why God had permitted such calamity to fall upon him. Revelation comes by way of the Holy Spirit as God ministers to each. As Job proclaimed, *"I know that You can do everything, And that no purpose of Yours can be withheld from You." (Job 42:2 NKJV)**

The details in Genesis have been shown to be chronologically accurate and has served humanity throughout the ages. Does it really matter for our continued reverence to the Almighty how a person interprets it? It most certainly does not!

How much "natural time" was there between Genesis 1 and Genesis 2? This is said to have occurred all in one day. But we are speaking of a God day in which time is nonexistent, a day in which much can supernaturally occur. This could represent a very long time for man, as I explained earlier.

Each of the six days in Genesis is described as fitting within the time frame of "evening and the morning." The seventh day is not described as within this frame of time; *"Thus the heavens and the earth, and all the host of them,* *were finished. And on the seventh day God ended His work which He had done, and He rested on the seventh day from all His work which He had done. Then God blessed the seventh day and sanctified it, because in it He rested from all His work which God had created and made."* (Genesis 2:1-3 NKJV)* This would imply that the day of rest for God is still on, while our natural days have continued.

In Genesis 1:28, God says, "Be fruitful and multiply; fill the earth and subdue it; have dominion over the fish of the sea, over the birds of the air, and over every living thing that moves on the earth." Was this meant for Adam? Was Adam not confined to the Garden of Eden?

Genesis was written so that it would make sense to both ancient and present day man. Only those who refute the existence of God have a problem with it. The entire Bible was written to traverse time and generations. Each time a person reads it, there is a different revelation. It is truly an incredible book.

There are revelations in Genesis which could only have been known by way of supernatural revelation or through the actual experience of the writer. Take for example the snake that tempted Eve. According to Genesis, this snake had legs. Paleontologists claim snakes evolved from lizards some 100 to 130 million years ago during the end of the Cretaceous Period. That is to say that snakes lost their legs 100 to 130 million years ago. God cursed the snake that decieved Eve by making the snake family legless, making them have to crawl on their belly. God turned the switch for the leg gene off. *"So the LORD God said to the serpent: 'Because you have done this, You are cursed more than all cattle, And more than every beast of the field; On your belly you shall go, And you shall eat dust All the days of your life.'"* (Genesis 3:14 NKJV)*

How could the writer of Genesis have known that snakes had legs at one time and that they lost them? This was a first-hand experience according to Genesis. We know from the study of snakes that snakes like the boa have tiny claws on the sides of the cloaca that are remnants of legs, but how would the writer of Genesis have known?

There is sufficient evidence that we were specifically designed by the creator God for a very special purpose: to reside ultimately in His perfect kingdom. God could have multiple kingdoms if He so desired since the whole cosmos is His domain. We must either accept Him or reject Him and accept the consequences of our decision.

Could there have been other men besides Adam during or before him? And if there were, would it make a difference? It certainly would not. The same goes for the possibility of beings on other planets. Could there be other civilizations on other planets, and if there is, what difference would it make? God has given earth to man. *"The heaven, even the heavens, are the LORD's. But the earth He has given to the children of men." (Psalms 115:16 NKJV)**

As man seeks for water and other signs of life on other planets, some dread that this would prove that there is no God. On the contrary, this will only prove the manifest greatness of God. What we will find is that they have the same creator God as we do, just as every civilization has had on Earth since recorded history. If life is found on some distant planet, we will not have to doubt one word in the Judeo-Christian Bible.

God has a practice of selecting certain individuals for specific tasks in His overall plan. God chose Adam. Likewise, God chose Noah, and Abraham, and Isaac, and their descendants up through today. It was through His select that God made provisions for the entire world.

However, we interpret the Genesis account does not detract from God's great and marvelous plan. Each one of us needs to study and make certain of God's plan for our own lives. Our eternity depends on it.

Only the Judeo-Christian Bible has demonstrated the supernatural numerology, accurate prophesies, accurate description of the cosmos, accurate chronology, accurate revelations, and God's marvelous plan through the perfect life and person of Jesus Christ.

We need to know God for who He is: our great and awesome Creator. He is the originator of our destiny to perfection. *"The fear of the LORD is the beginning of wisdom, And the knowledge of the Holy One is understanding." (Proverbs 9:10 NKJV)**

Knowledge of the Holy One is knowledge of Jesus Christ, the anointed one, the Son of God, who is also described as the right hand of God. *"Indeed My hand has laid the foundation of the earth, And My right hand has stretched out the heavens; When I call to them, They stand up together." (Isaiah 48:13 NKJV)** This verse also bears witness of the triune nature of God. "When I call out to them, they stand up together" implies that there are at least two, and God the Father makes three. The two are identified as the hands of God.

Jesus is also revealed as the bearer of God's Holy name. *"Behold, the days are coming," says the LORD, "That I will raise to David a Branch of righteousness; A King shall reign and prosper, And execute judgment and righteousness in the earth. In His days Judah will be saved, And Israel will dwell safely; Now this is His name by which He will be called: THE LORD (YAHVEH) OUR RIGHTEOUSNESS." (Jeremiah 23:5–6 NKJV)**

In the King James Version of the Bible, "LORD" is used in place of the original word, which is Jehovah, or Yahveh, the name of God the Father, the name which Isaiah proclaims God will not share with anyone. *"I am the LORD, that is My name; And My glory I will not give to another, Nor My praise to carved images." (Isaiah 42:8 NKJV)** "My hand" and *"My right hand"* makes reference to interactive body parts which are synonymous with the Spirit and the Messiah.

This Jesus is not only special, but is also a part of the creator God, identified as His right hand, a critical part of His own being. The Bible claims that all things in the universe were created by God through Jesus Christ. In the Old Testament, Proverbs proclaims: *"From the beginning, before there was ever an earth. When there were no depths I was brought forth, when there were no fountains abounding with water. Before the mountains were settled, before the hills, I was brought forth; while as yet He had not made the earth or the fields, or the primal dust of the world. When He prepared the heavens, I was there, when He drew a circle on the face of the deep, when He established the clouds above, when He strengthened the fountains of the deep, when He assigned to the sea its limit, so that the waters would not transgress His command, when He marked out the foundations of the earth, then I was beside Him as a master craftsman." (Proverbs 8:22–30 NKJV)**

In John we find: *"In the beginning was the Word, and the Word was with God, and the Word was God. He was in the beginning with God. All things were made through Him, and without Him nothing was made that was made." (John 1:1–3 NKJV)**

Colossians also mentions the creation through Christ Jesus. *"He has delivered us from the power of darkness and* *conveyed us into the kingdom of the Son of His love, in whom we have redemption through His blood, the forgiveness of sins. He is the image of the invisible God, the firstborn over all creation. For by Him all things were created that are in heaven and that are on earth, visible and invisible, whether thrones or dominions or principalities or powers. All things were created through Him and for Him. And He is before all things, and in Him all things consist. And He is the head of the body, the church, who is the beginning, the firstborn from the dead, that in all things He may have the preeminence." (Colossians 1:13–18 NKJV)**

Chapter 17

1. In the book of _____, we learn that God made man.

2. Genesis is written so that it would make _____ to both ancient and present man.

3. We must either accept Him or reject Him and accept the _____ of our decision.

4. God has a practice of _____ certain individuals for specific tasks in His overall plan.

5. The Bible claims that all things in the _____ were created by God through Jesus Christ.

6. Jesus is also revealed as the _____ of God's very name.

Answers: Genesis, sense, consequences, selecting, universe, bearer

Chapter Eighteen

Destructive Doctrine

Of all of the destructive doctrines ever devised by man, there is probably none worse than the doctrine of creation through evolution. When confronted with the doctrine of creation through evolution, a person must ask how this doctrine actually affects us.

This doctrine of creation through evolution, as benign as some suppose it to be, nullifies the need for believing in a creator God and because of this, is the most destructive doctrine to mankind of all false doctrines that exist today.

Jesus in describing Himself stated: *"I am the door. If anyone enters by Me, he will be saved, and will go in and out and find pasture. The thief does not come except to steal, and to kill, and to destroy. I have come that they may have life, and that they may have it more abundantly." (John 10:9–10 NKJV)* *

The doctrine of creation through evolution destroys the need to believe in a creator God and provides an excuse as to why one does not need to believe, in effect stealing the individual's salvation. While the doctrine of creation through evolution sounds rational, it is highly disputed and not accepted by many scientists. Common Descent or Common Creator is a matter of choice, not science.

There are many flaws in the doctrine of creation through evolution which many people disregard. Darwin predicted that many transitional forms would be found. Yet, to this day, both the gradual pattern of change and lineage is missing from the fossil record. That there is great diversity among the species is true, but diversity does not constitute evidence for transitional forms.

Take the dog, Canis lupus, for example. A great diversity has been bred from canine stock in the last couple of centuries. However, genetic diversity does not provide proof for creation through evolution.

While some geneticists are re-categorizing the many breeds as different species to bolster their creation through evolution argument, it is well accepted that these are different breeds of the same species. Left alone, they would interbreed and revert back to the wild genome.

There are many single-cell life forms but virtually no forms of life consisting of two or three cells. If creation actually occurred through evolution, there would be many such transitional forms.

All species are capable of great diversity and innumerable traits. We know this to be a fact. Humans have been doing selective breeding of animals since recorded history. Selective breeding can also be influenced by the environment and isolation. Such changes and findings, however, do not prove creation through evolution. The records found are scant and are only demonstrating diversity and not creation through evolution.

As I discussed earlier in the book, new species are the result of multiple beneficial genetic changes occurring simultaneously, not single changes occurring sporadically over millions of years, i.e. the giraffe. Organisms that are able to breed and produce like kind are considered to be of the same species. If a gene transfer is performed and the species can still interbreed and produce like kind, it would still be the same species, regardless what someone designates it to be.

We know that the great majority of random genetic changes are detrimental to the species and not beneficial, leading to the destruction of the organism. Selective gene transfer can result in a viable organism because it is selected to produce a minor noncritical trait at a specific site on the genome. This generally results in a variant trait in the species. Multiple gene transferring or the transfer of a critical gene can result in a truly new species. Such engineering is more involved and requires greater knowledge of the ramifications of the transfer. The complexity demonstrates the impossibility of creation, occurring spontaneously through evolution and affirms the necessity of a creative designer.

Diversity is an adaptive mechanism encoded into the genetic map of the species. Diversity is caused to be expressed by selective breeding. Expression of previously unrevealed genetic types does not make for evolution of new species. The similarity between species implies a common intelligent designer and not evolution.

The genes for diversity are encoded so as to fit into the genetic architecture of the species for optimized function and survival. A new species requires major architectural modifications to fit together properly to enable species survival.

Darwin looked at species diversity and said, "This explains the origin of the species," without fully considering the complex changes involved in the creation of a new species. A greater understanding of the complexities involved would have caused Darwin to have considered creation through evolution impossible as he admitted in his book *On the Origin of Species by Means of Natural Selection.*

The age of the earth is irrelevant to the Genesis account of creation since the creation of heaven and earth was prior to the Genesis story. *"In the beginning God created the heavens and the earth. The earth was without form, and void; and darkness was on the face of the deep. And the Spirit of God was hovering over the face of the waters.Then God said, 'Let there be light'; and there was light. And God saw the light that it was good; and God divided the light from the darkness. God called the light Day, and the darkness He called Night. So the evening and the morning were the first day."(Genesis 1:1-5 NKJV)**

The aging of the earth and universe is based on assumptions and not on strict science. Scientist do not know the effect on time should the expansion of the universe have occurred at a million or a billion times faster than the speed of light, a finding which was previously thought to be impossible but which seems now more probable than previously.

We constantly have to correct our calculations as new information is learned. Even dinosaurs that had been previously identified have had to be re-categorized as youngsters of another known species. Planet vegetation and specific elemental content may have been very different in the past grossly distorting the references used.

Radiometric dating requires the acceptance of multiple assumptions which can create major errors in dating. It assumes that the rate of decay remains constant for billions of years of earth's history, that the material tested had zero content of the breakdown or daughter element to begin with and that no entry or escape occurred of either the initial or the daughter elements.

Neutron bombardment by supernova explosions which are believed to have occurred multiple times in the past billion years of the earth's history rapidly increases rates of radiometric material decay. Water washing out uranium salts, magma absorbing argon, a decay product, all of these processes can falsely increase age calculations.[19]

Entropy, the second law in thermodynamics, laws on which all other physical laws depend, that is, that all things in the universe left alone become less organized, is violated by creation through evolution.

The law of maximum entropy production, that entropy will select the path or paths that minimize the potential or maximize the entropy at the fastest rate – in other words select the fastest and easiest way to disperse energy – is violated by creation through evolution.

Life from life, the Law of Biogenesis, a scientific fact, and applicable to all life forms on Earth is violated by creation through evolution.

Most spontaneous genetic changes are detrimental to the species. Rather than moving to a more ideal species form, species are becoming less ideal for the environmental changes and are dying off at a rapid rate.

As stated earlier, sexually reproducing species – of which there are millions – require that each sex evolve in the same manner and at the same time. This intricately complex simultaneous co-evolution would have to occur millions of times over for all obligate co-dependent organisms to survive and reproduce. This process occurring spontaneously is not only highly improbable but impossible.

Creation by God is a supernatural event and entails expert manipulation and design. The potentials are enormous as can be seen by the vast varieties of species in nature. Co-dependant species are created simultaneously so that propagation of the species is facilitated. Gene variation permits divergence which facilitates adaptation for survival of the species.

Without knowledgeable purposeful design, creation would not be possible. The adaptation abilities of each species permits great diversity for enhanced survival. Without such, life would have eventually disappeared.

Despite the arguments, the doctrine of creation through evolution has gained over the creation-by-God doctrine. This is partially due to ignorance and the refusal to accept that God could actually be a reality. Many feel they have no option but to accept the creation through evolution since without God there is no other reasonable explanation for creation.

There is a demonic force behind the doctrine of cre-ation through evolution, it is bent on our destruction. This has led and contributed to the decline in morals and rise in lawlessness that now exist around the world and that will ultimately lead to the demise of those who do not rely on the saving grace of God.

It is not religion that has caused all of the many dis-putes that we see in the world. It is the *perversion* of religion that has caused division and strife. Imagine what the world would be like if everyone practiced the love principle as required by Christ. Instead, we have adopted demonic principles and doctrines that have caused strife and hatred which are leading us to our doom. The principles, practices, and doctrines are orchestrated by Satan to destroy mankind.

The doctrine of creation through evolution tells us we are the product of blind random chemical reactions formed by chance and that we are no different than the animals we consider inferior. Our closest relative relies on brute strength and swings from trees. We have no help and no hope. The odds are stacked up against us.

The doctrine of creation through evolution teaches that we have no purpose or reason for our being and that we have a meaningless existence on a small and insignificant planet with ultimate destruction as our destiny. Our lives require that we defeat the competition in our survival of the fittest mode of existence. No one truly matters but oneself.

The doctrine of creation through evolution teaches us that morals are not made by an all-loving God but by each individual according to their own pleasures and displeasures. We are entitled to whatever we can get or get away with, since when it is all over there is nothing more. There is no need for fellowship, no accountability, and no need to care. We can do what we want, when we want, for as long as we want, for as long as we can get away with it. It is all by chance, and you only get one life so make the best of it.

On the contrary, the Christian creation by God doctrine tells us we are a special creation of a good and all-powerful loving God. It tells us that we were created in His image, a high point of His creation, with the capacity to think and to choose from right and wrong. He has given us the ability to experience emotions, to love and have passion, and to adore and to worship, setting us above all life forms. And if we choose to do right, He rewards us, blessing our walk and our loved ones.

The Christian creation-by-God doctrine teaches that God wants to bless us a thousand times more than to punish us for our disobedience. *"...For I, the LORD your God, am a jealous God, visiting the iniquity of the fathers upon the children to the third and fourth generations of those who hate Me, but showing mercy to thousands, to those who love Me and keep My commandments."* (Exodus 20:5–6 NKJV)*

The Christian creation-by-God doctrine teaches that we differ from all the animals not simply in kind but in selection, chosen of God for a special and specific purpose, cared for and destined to be ministered to by the angels, as it is written: *"Are they not all ministering spirits sent forth to minister for those who will inherit salvation?"* (Hebrews 1:14 NKJV)*

The Christian creation-by-God doctrine teaches us that God not only masterminded our individual uniqueness but also made us uniquely special. The book of Psalms declares: *"For You formed my inward parts; You covered me in my mother's womb. I will praise You, for I am fearfully and wonderfully made; Marvelous are Your works, and that my soul knows very well. My frame was not hidden from You, when I was made in secret, and skillfully wrought in the lowest parts of the earth. Your eyes saw my substance, being yet unformed. And in Your book they all were written, the days fashioned for me, When as yet there were none of them."* (Psalms 139:13–16 NKJV)*

The Christian creation-by-God doctrine teaches that it isn't only significant that He created us, but also that we are important to Him, as it is written: *"When I consider Your heavens, the work of Your fingers, The moon and the stars, which You have ordained, what is man that You are mindful of him, and the son of man that You visit him? For You have made him a little lower than the angels, and You have crowned him with glory and honor. You have made him to have dominion over the works of Your hands; You have put all things under his feet, all sheep and oxen even the beasts of the field, the birds of the air, and the fish of the sea that pass through the paths of the seas. O LORD, our Lord, How excellent is Your name in all the earth!" (Psalms 8:3–9 NKJV)**

Beyond this, it teaches us that, we are not just important to Him but that He also loves us: *"For God so loved the world that He gave His only begotten Son, that whoever believes in Him should not perish but have everlasting life. For God did not send His Son into the world to condemn the world, but that the world through Him might be saved." (John 3:16–17 NKJV)**

The Christian creation-by-God doctrine not only demonstrates that God loves us, but it also assures us that we will be with Him even after death. *"But I do not want you to be ignorant, brethren, concerning those who have fallen asleep, lest you sorrow as others who have no hope. For if we believe that Jesus died and rose again, even so God will bring with Him those who sleep in Jesus. For this we say to you by the word of the Lord, that we who are alive and remain until the coming of the Lord will by no means precede those who are asleep. For the Lord Himself will descend from heaven with a shout, with the voice of an archangel, and with the trumpet of God. And the dead in Christ will rise first. Then we who are alive and remain shall* be caught up together with them in the clouds to meet the Lord in the air. And thus we shall always be with the Lord. Therefore comfort one another with these words." (1 Thessalonians 4:13–18 NKJV)*

The Christian creation-by-God doctrine teaches that despite not having access to any laws of God, all people are born into this world with a conviction of God's standards, defined as "the law written in their hearts" by which they will be judged even if they have never heard of God or the Gospel of Jesus. *"For there is no partiality with God. For as many as have sinned without law will also perish without law, and as many as have sinned in the law will be judged by the law (for not the hearers of the law are just in the sight of God, but the doers of the law will be justified; for when Gentiles, who do not have the law, by nature do the things in the law, these, although not having the law, are a law to themselves, who show the work of the law written in their hearts, their conscience also bearing witness, and between themselves their thoughts accusing or else excusing them) in the day when God will judge the secrets of men by Jesus Christ, according to my gospel."* (Romans 2:11–16 NKJV)*

The Christian creation-by-God doctrine offers encouragement, protection, reassurance, love, and hope, unlike any doctrine that man has devised. *"And we know that all things work together for good to those who love God, to those who are the called according to His purpose. For whom He foreknew, He also predestined to be conformed to the image of His Son, that He might be the firstborn among many brethren. Moreover whom He predestined, these He also called; whom He called, these He also justified; and whom He justified, these He also glorified. What then shall we say to these things? If God is for us, who can be against us? He who did not spare His own Son, but delivered Him up* *for us all, how shall He not with Him also freely give us all things?" (Romans 8:28–32 NKJV)**

As humans, we need to know that we are loved. We need to have a sense of value to produce endorphins or feel good hormones. Without a good self-esteem, humans are self-destructive and destructive to others. Bitterness and uncaring attitudes set in which disrupt our organ systems, inducing disease and death.

Contrary to the doctrine of creation through evolution and its mode of operating of survival of the fittest, the creation by God mode requires that we love and help one another. We love and serve God by loving and serving each other. The evolution concept creates contention and adversity while creation creates harmony and family.

Contention is contrary to what the Bible declares that God wants for us and plays into what the Bible declares as to what God's enemies want. If I were in error, I would rather be in error on God's side than on God's enemy's side, for only God offers to reward us. The alternative provides only curses and destruction.

Religions that buy into theistic evolution, that God used evolution to bring about creation, deny the supernatural omnipotence of God and the veracity of His word. They make God no more a god than the wood and stones of the pagan gods and expose themselves to the wrath and curses intended for the unbeliever.

The Scriptures state that such false teachings will bring about the wrath of God in due time. *"But there were also false prophets among the people, even as there will be false teachers among you, who will secretly bring in destructive heresies, even denying the Lord who bought* *them, and bring on themselves swift destruction. And many will follow their destructive ways, because of whom the way of truth will be blasphemed. By covetousness they will exploit you with deceptive words; for a long time their judgment has not been idle, and their destruction does not slumber." (2 Peter 2:1–3 NKJV)**

A supernatural God cannot be explained by natural means. Religious leaders have gotten caught up in the scientists' attempt to explain supernatural events by natural means. It is utterly impossible to do so since they are completely different dimensions, a natural dimension which is bound by natural laws and God's dimension which is outside of the laws of nature.

Religious leaders who accept the scientists' explanation must either abandon their faith – since their god is not the God of the Bible – or deny the scientist explanation and accept the omnipotence of God and the supernatural events spoken of in the Bible.

Chapter 18

1. Of all of the _____ doctrines ever devised by man, there is probably none worse than the doctrine of creation through evolution.

2. Without a good self-_____, humans are self-destructive and destructive to others; bitterness and uncaring attitudes set in which disrupt our organ systems inducing disease and death.

3. The Christian creation-by-God doctrine offers encouragement, protection, _____, love, and hope unlike any doctrine that man has devised.

4. The Christian creation-by-God doctrine not only demonstrates that God loves us, but it also _____ us that we will be with Him even after death.

5. Religions that buy into _____ evolution, that God used evolution to bring about creation, deny the supernatural omnipotence of God and the veracity of His word.

6. A supernatural God cannot be explained by _____ means.

Answers: destructive, esteem, reassurance, assures, theistic, natural

Chapter Nineteen

Acquiring an Ideal Body

God promises those, who repent, accept Yahshua's sacrifice, and emulate Him, the gift of eternal life. I have discussed previously how our body will be transformed into a glorified, perfected body — an ideal body— like the body of Yahshua. The Bible in various places in the Old and New Testament documents the resurrection of the dead and their transformation, along with the living at the time of His return. We find this in several passages of the Bible.

In Daniel: *"At that time Michael shall stand up, The great prince who stands watch over the sons of your people; And there shall be a time of trouble, Such as never was since there was a nation, Even to that time. And at that time your people shall be delivered, everyone who is found written in the book. And many of those who sleep in the dust of the earth shall awake, some to everlasting life, some to shame and everlasting contempt. Those who are wise shall shine like the brightness of the firmament, and those who turn many to righteousness like the stars forever and ever."* (Daniel 12:1–3 NKJV)*

In 1ˢᵗ Thessalonians: *"For this we say to you by the word of the Lord, that we who are alive and remain until the coming of the Lord will by no means precede those who are asleep. For the Lord Himself will descend from heaven with a shout, with the voice of an archangel, and with the trumpet of God. And the dead in Christ will rise first. Then we who are alive and remain shall be caught up together with them* in the clouds to meet the Lord in the air. And thus we shall always be with the Lord."(1 Thessalonians 4:15–17 NKJV)*

In Titus: "Looking for the blessed hope and glorious appearing of our great God and Savior Jesus Christ, who gave Himself for us, that He might redeem us from every lawless deed and purify for Himself His own special people, zealous for good works." (Titus 2:13–14 NKJV)*

In Revelation: " 'And behold, I am coming quickly, and My reward is with Me, to give to everyone according to his work. I am the Alpha and the Omega, the Beginning and the End, the First and the Last.' Blessed are those who do His commandments that they may have the right to the tree of life, and may enter through the gates into the city." (Revelation 22:12–14 NKJV)*

When God placed Adam in the Garden of Eden, He placed him there to live in paradise for as long as Adam complied with God's rule of not eating from the Tree of Knowledge of Good and Evil. Did God not know that Adam would not comply? Did God not know that Adam's mate would be enticed by the serpent and eat of the Tree of Knowledge of Good and Evil? God had to have known.

When God came looking for Adam, did He not know what they had done? Did God not tell the serpent that the seed of woman would crush his head? Was not God's plan already in place? God had to have known. He is omniscient. God's purpose for placing the Tree of Knowledge of Good and Evil was so that Adam would be tempted so that he would choose his own fate and the fate of his progeny. The Tree of Life was also there in the Garden of Eden so that Adam could know that eternal life was also an option if he were to be obedient.

These are the same options that each one of us has today. We can choose obedience and receive the gift of etenal life, or we can choose disobedience and be denied entry to God's eternal paradise, basically, the same options Adam and Eve were given.

The Garden of Eden was a type of eternal paradise. The difference between the Garden of Eden and God's final paradise is the presence of God. In the eternal paradise, God will dwell with man. That is why man would have to be perfect, perfected through the sacrifice of Yahshua, God's Messiah.

Some people regard this as something we can hope for, but the Bible clearly states that this is something that we can know. For it states: *"I write these things to you who believe in the name of the Son of God so that you may know that you have eternal life." (1 John 5:13 NKJV)** The word that is used here is "know" not "hope," thus we can know that we have eternal life if we believe in the Son.

We, therefore, are given a guarantee that if we obey God's Word, accept the sacrifice of His Son, and become like His Son, we will, at His return, be transformed like the glorified ideal body of Jesus Christ to abide forever in God's perfect Holy Kingdom. It is written,*"Beloved, now we are children of God; and it has not yet been revealed what we shall be, but we know that when He is revealed, we shall be like Him, for we shall see Him as He is." (1st John 3:2 NKJV)**

Someone may say that it does not say that you have to become like Jesus, but the fact is that the word believe in Hebrew, "aman, אמן" has the same root as "amen" and is a word of affirmation. It means to conform, to have assurance, to be faithful. In other words, you cannot say that you believe in something and act like something else.

Therefore, if you say you believe in Yahshua, you must be like Yahshua.

The peace of knowing Yahshua is the peace of knowing you will be taken care of for all eternity. There is no greater peace, regardless of the adversity that you may be facing. This is God's promise, a promise you can depend on and a promise made by the Creator of the universe. You can be sure that there is no greater backing.

May this assurance give you peace and strength to continue your walk in life, knowing that you are not alone but that He is with you, preparing the way and guiding you, watching and waiting, and providing for whatever you have need of.

Some of you may be at the end of your worldly tour and are afraid, but there is nothing to fear for the glory that is before you is many times more glorious than the past that you will be leaving behind. God will take care of the loved ones that you leave behind. There is nothing to worry about for His promises are eternal. Leave it all to Him. God is not interested in preserving you for this world – He is interested in preparing you for the next. So be joyful and glorify God.

Chapter 19

1. God _____ those, who repent, accept Yahshua's sacrifice, and emulate Him, the gift of eternal life.

2. The Bible in various places in the Old and New Testament documents the _____ of the dead and their transformation along with the living at the time of Yashua's return.

3. Some people regard this as something we can hope for, but the Bible clearly states that this is something that we can _____.

4. We, therefore, are given a _____ that if we obey God's Word, accept the sacrifice of His son, and become like His son, we will, at His return, be transformed into a body like the glorified ideal body of Yahshua.

5. To abide _____ in God's Holy perfect Kingdom.

6. God is not interested in _____ you for this world – He is interested in preparing you for the next. So be joyful and glorify God.

Answers: promises, resurrection, know, guarantee, forever, preserving

Chapter Twenty

Our Earthly Body

Some persons may have purchased this book, thinking that it is only a book about our natural body. The preceding chapters do have implications on our earthly existence. However, it is now that I believe some general knowledge on health issues that affect all of us is in order. In this last chapter, I will share current knowledge useful in optimizing one's health.

The advice in this chapter is not intended to treat any disease state and should only be undertaken with the guidance and advice of your personal physician.

First of all, I want to stress that the gold standard continues to be diet and exercise. The old adage that we are what we eat is basically true. A health practitioner can only guide you. You are the one that gets to choose what you eat and how much, whether you walk or ride, or take the elevator or the stairs. Choosing to expend energy rather than to take the lazy approach is healthful and should be a consistent and conscious effort.

Like almost anything in our lives, healthful living habits require discipline. This is something most of us lack and need to work on. Disciplining oneself to eat right takes as much fortitude and willpower as keeping a fast; the more or longer you do it, the easier it becomes. Your dietary habits should be beneficial, rational, and permanent – a way of living.

Moderate exercise, if you can safely do it, is excellent. When exercising for health, never work yourself to the point of pain or exhaustion, as this is your body warning you that you are exceeding the body's limit. Rather, increase your exercise as your tolerance increases. Give yourself adequate time between exercising for your body to recuperate, and remember that rest is as important as exercise. Try and assure that you get adequate sleep. Seven hours a night is probably optimal unless you have been deprived of sleep for some time and require additional sleep to catch up.

Taking drugs to induce sleep produces unnatural sleep which can make you feel tired and prone to falling asleep during waketime hours. This is hazardous if performing anything particularly dangerous, such as driving a motor vehicle. A practice that can help one stay awake during such times is sucking on ice. The cold ice in your mouth increases blood flow to the brain which makes you more alert. It also may help burn additional calories.

Hormonal issues especially in older individuals can cause anxiety and sleep problems. These issues are often overlooked. Such problems should be investigated by a qualified healthcare provider.

Your immune system is revitalized while you sleep. It does not have to compete with the active musculoskeletal system during this time, and the peptide hormones produced while you sleep, stimulate the immune system. This is why patients with autoimmune disorders wake up with more pain in the mornings. Their immune system is stronger in the early morning hours upon arising from sleep. If you deprive yourself of sleep, your immune system will be impaired, and you will be more susceptible to illness.

It is important to realize that our bodies function on a circadian rhythm. That is, our hormonal, gastrointestinal, and brain functions maintain a time-sensitive repetitive routine that is established by the sleep/wake cycle that we keep. Repetitive changes in our sleep/wake cycle can be extremely detrimental to this circadian rhythm. This can lead to altered function and disease. Keep a routine that supports this circadian rythm to optimize your well-being.

Exercise to counter the effects of gravity on your body when possible with spinal stretching exercises such as pull-ups or pulling weights down rather than lifting heavy objects that compress your spine. Keeping your bones strong and preserving the joint spaces will benefit every organ system in your body.

Doing heavy overhead weight lifting into old age increases the neck and shoulder angle, compresses the spine and abdominal organs, and can cause hernias and hemorrhoids to develop. The increased neck and shoulder angle makes the neck seem longer and detracts from a person's attractiveness.

Consumption of large amounts of vegetables and fruits is important for providing the minerals for strong bones and alkalinizing the body. This prevents calcium from leaching out of the bones and helps maintain strong bones. The worst enemy to a weakened musculoskeletal system as you age is gravity and undue stress. Do what you can to avoid their effects. Stretching and decompression exercises and regular alignment procedures is a good practice.

Do what you can to avoid stress. The stress hor-mones are catabolic. They tear you down and cause you to age faster. Avoid substances or situations wherein you are likely to experience stress. Learn to stay calm and not overreact to any situation. Remember that it is not what you experience but rather how you receive the experience that determines the production of these hormones.

Drink plenty of fluids, unless you have heart or kidney problems. Individuals with heart or kidney problems or those who are taking medications should consult their physician as to how much fluids they should consume and how much exercise they can safely perform. When you feel your best, weigh yourself on a reliable scale. A sudden gain or loss in weight could be an indicator that you need fluids (weight down) or have too much fluid (weight up).

As a general rule regarding fluids, individuals with normal kidneys and heart function should take in half of their weight in ounces on a daily basis. To obtain your optimal fluid intake, divide your weight by two and multiply this by the number of hours you are normally awake. This amount will indicate the number of ounces of water that you will require on a given day.

For example, if an individual weighs 130 pounds and is awake 16 hours a day, they should consume 65 ounces divided by 16 or 4 ounces per hour. Distributing one's water intake over the entire day is more beneficial than drinking large amounts at once because it is better distributed and not rapidly eliminated by the body. A simplified rule is to drink about a cup of drinking water per wake hour per day. Drinking water with minerals is better than distilled water, which lacks minerals and is less beneficial.

Your body acclimates to the temperature and humidity in the environment. An individual can be mildly dehydrated and not feel that there is anything wrong. This is important because the increased viscosity or thickness of the blood, due to the reduced fluid volume, can increase clotting risk and set an individual up for a heart attack or stroke. Maintaining good hydration is very important.

Diet is most important, and fresh foods are best. Preservatives, food additives, colorings, artificial sweeteners, simple sugars, animal fats, and refined foods should definitely be avoided. A diet high in vegetables and fruits with some lean meat and fish is preferable. Low-calorie, high-nutrition should be the routine. Reducing caloric intake with high-nutrient foods has been shown to be beneficial for slowing aging and reducing inflammation, arthritis, cancer, and cardiovascular diseases. Eating these foods with olive oil and other cold-press vegetable oils high in omega-3 fatty acids helps provide optimum function. Some meat is necessary for adequate B12 and carnitine consumption. These vital nutrients are absent in purely vegan diets. Vegetarians should consume some eggs to assure adequate B12 and carnitine intake.

Animal fat is not to be eaten. In the book of Leviticus God instructs Moses: *"The LORD said to Moses, 'Say to the Israelites: "Do not eat any of the fat of cattle, sheep or goats. The fat of an animal found dead or torn by wild animals may be used for any other purpose, but you must not eat it." (Leviticus 7:22–25 NKJV)**

We know today that the consumption of animal fat has detrimental effects on the body and is associated with arteriosclerosis, inflammatory diseases, heart attacks, cancers, and strokes. Such advice given over 3,500 years ago is an incredible revelation of the omniscience of Almighty God.

The first experiment in recorded history is found in the book of Daniel where Daniel is asked to eat sacrificial meats and the delicacies from the king's fare. Daniel refuses and instead requests to be permitted to consume vegetables and water. Daniel's caretaker was afraid that Daniel would appear undernourished but permitted Daniel and his friends to consume only vegetables and water. Ten days later, he found that Daniel and his friends appeared healthier than the men permitted to eat the meats and delicacies that Daniel and his friends had refused. *"But Daniel purposed in his heart that he would not defile himself with the portion of the king's delicacies, nor with the wine which he drank; therefore he requested of the chief of the eunuchs that he might not defile himself. Now God had brought Daniel into the favor and goodwill of the chief of the eunuchs. And the chief of the eunuchs said to Daniel, 'I fear my lord the king, who has appointed your food and drink. For why should he see your faces looking worse than the young men who are your age? Then you would endanger my head before the king.' So Daniel said to the steward whom the chief of the eunuchs had set over Daniel, Hananiah, Mishael, and Azariah, 'Please test your servants for ten days, and let them give us vegetables to eat and water to drink. Then let our appearance be examined before you, and the appearance of the young men who eat the portion of the king's delicacies; and as you see fit, so deal with your servants.' So he consented with them in this matter, and tested them in ten days. And at the end of ten days their features appeared better and fatter in flesh than all the young men who ate the portion of the king's delicacies. Thus the steward took away their portion of delicacies and the wine that they were to drink, and gave them vegetables."* (Daniel 1:8–16 NKJV)**

Some use this "first" experiment to argue in favor of a purely vegan diet. But the fact is that it was only for 10 days and not sufficiently long enough for any deficiency to develop. In Israel, Daniel would have consumed meat and would have adequate stores of B12 and carnitine to prevent any signs of deficiency from developing over 10 days. Human teeth indicate humans are omnivorous, that is, they were made to consume vegetables and meat.

This self-imposed diet that Daniel requested is frequently called the Daniel fast, suggesting this to be a sacrificial-type diet. This diet with a small addition of some lean meat or eggs is a good all-around diet to consume on an ongoing basis. Unfortunately, all too often, people consume these meals with fatty cream-based dressings which nullify the benefit. Using olive oil or a puree of vegetables or fruit can enhance the flavor and augment the benefit.

As stated, a diet high in a variety of colorful raw vegetables and fruits provides plenty of calcium and minerals. This helps alkalinize the body which strengthens the bones and helps maintain enzyme function, reducing cancer risk and improving circulation and hormone function

Such diets provide high free-radical consumption and protection from oxidative stress. Green leafy vegetables are high in B vitamins and folic acid, which are vital for various metabolic functions and proper detoxification. Young plants and seeds are high in enzymes and provide additional benefits to digestion.

A problem many individuals have which is more prevalent among the elderly is poor dentition. Others fail to chew their food adequately enough to optimize digestion. In such cases, juicing is preferable to optimize nutrient acquisition.

Overcooking of vegetables should be avoided. Mild steaming is preferable and helps preserve the nutritional content. When possible, eat the vegetables raw. A good example is okra. The seeds in okra are high in enzymes, and their consumption is most beneficial when eaten raw. Instead, we cook or fry them and destroy their enzymes. Okras are slimy when cooked because of their high enzyme content. Proteolytic enzymes are reported to play a role in destruction of malignant cells, thinning blood mucous, and destroying debris in the blood. These functions are impaired by acidity which deactivates proteolytic enzymes. Pureed raw okras are excellent for adding to vegetable juices, smoothies or dips.

Assuring daily bowel movements is important. A newborn infant has a bowel movement after each meal. Having a bowel movement after eating is a normal reflex reaction that is lost due to our inhibitions and dietary habits. A person should have a minimum of one or two bowel movements per day. Anything less is unacceptable. An individual eliminates many toxins, metabolites, and hormones from their body in the stool. These can be reabsorbed from the intestine if they are present for too long and can accumulate in tissues. The hormonal increase can have secondary effects on the individual and can provoke sex-organ problems like fibrocystic breast disease, uterine fibroids or enlargement, dysfunctional uterine bleeding, prostatic enlargement, or cancers. In fact, constipation is a common problem in cancer patients even prior to their taking pain medications that impair bowel motility, a problem that is frequently overlooked.

Foul stools are an indicator of impaired digestion and overgrowth of deleterious bacteria, the higher the level of these aromatic hydrocarbons responsible for the malodorous stool, the higher the risk of colon cancer. It is important to pay attention to the odor, color, frequency, and firmness of your bowel movements.

Halatosis, or bad breath, is frequently due to malodorous volatile hydrocarbons arising from the gastrointestinal track that cross into the blood and are breathed out through the lungs. In such cases, supplementing with digestive enzymes and beneficial bacteria or probiotics, to resolve these problems may be necessary.

A common and growing problem in the world today is the toxicities with which we are burdened with. Heavy metals and organic pollutants are accumulating in the environment and in life forms at a rapid rate. The effects of the bio-accumulation of these agents are not fully understood. The increase body burden of toxins may be why we are seeing increases in cancers and developmental and degenerative diseases in all age groups.

One problem is the increased demands on nutrient cofactors. With higher toxic burden, it is increasingly more important that an individual consume large amounts of vegetables high in nutrient cofactors and fiber. Increasing intestinal motility is important in eliminating toxicities. Supplementing with nutrients that supports the individual's ability to detoxify is especially valuable in such individuals.

A toxin's effect on an individual increases the toxicity effects of other toxins. For example, low-level lead and low-level mercury can be more toxic than either metal given alone at higher doses. That is, the LD50 (amount of lead that will kill 50% of individuals) and the LD50 (amount of mercury that will kill 50% of individuals), when given together, will kill 100% of individuals. This exponential effect of combined toxicities is routinely seen with numerous toxins.

Electrical pollutants which have increased a million-fold over the past 10 years likewise augment the toxic effects of biological toxins. It is generally an accepted fact that the more toxic an individual is the more susceptible the individual is to the effects of radiation and electrical pollutants.

In my experience, cancer patients and patients with immune disorders routinely have higher levels of toxicities. Avoiding disease is why it is important that individuals constantly work on reducing their toxic burden by using detoxifying regimens, diet, and by increasing their bodily functions. Cancer cells appear to be cells struggling to survive in a toxic environment. Eliminating or reducing the toxic burden is frequently ignored in cancer therapy yet should be a priority in these patients.

It is important for individuals to check around their homes to determine if they could be getting exposed to excessive electrical pollution. Eliminating this exposure is one way of reducing ones toxic burden. Whether it is by moving away from high-tension cables or moving their bed away from high-electromagnetic radiation and electric fields, any reduction in such exposure could have major implications to a person's well-being.

A toxic individual would benefit from supplementing their diet with nutrients that support detoxification and mitochondrial function. Mitochondria are the organelles in each cell that are responsible for energy production and are the target of many toxins. As the cell loses mitochondria, cell survival diminishes.

Low level toxicity should not be ignored, especially if there is disease present. Disease is an indication that the individual is already decompensating. Alleviating the toxic burden supports the body's ability to heal.

Lead (Pb) toxicity is a common cause of kidney failure in the United States.[20] Low level lead can contribute to the onset and rapidity of kidney damage in patients with renal impairment due to diabetes or hypertension. Reducing lead burden could help improve and maintain optimum renal function.

There are various laboratories and clinics around the United States that provide testing and treatments for individuals suffering from toxicity-related problems. Oftentimes, toxic burden is what prevents an individual from recovering.

Industry and certain individuals supported by industry would downplay the potential detrimental effects of exposure to biological toxins. Safe levels of exposure are held at a strict level when individual susceptability dictates that any level can be dangerous to a particular individual.

Individuals can have different tolerance levels. Those who advocate "no effect" to particular levels and label themselves as "consumer advocates" are actual wolves in sheeps clothing. One only need look at who is supporting them to know where they are coming from. If they have websites, look at who is advertising on their sites. No doubt, their motives are monetary.... *"For the love of money is a root of all kinds of evil, for which some have strayed from the faith in their greediness, and pierced themselves through with many sorrows." (1st Timothy 6:10 NKJV)**

They and the companies who support them are unworthy of support or patronage. Their true motive is to downplay toxicity effects for industry and to limit health and testing for insurers to maximize profits. They claim certain expertise, but their only true expertise is in defamation and slander.

Like the creation through evolution dogma, they deny the complex nature of our being and ignore the destruction of life and societal problems their false doctines incite.

Toxic level implies a level which causes a detrimental effect on an individual. Detrimental effects may not be apparent until significant damage has occurred and hence may be discovered too late. There is, therefore, no "safe level" for a biological toxin that has no benefit.

A person's tolerance level is determined by the total sum of the individual's ability to deal with their toxic burden. An individual's prior exposure, their nutrient cofactor levels, hydration status, oxygenation status, methylation capacity, sulfation capacity, glutathione status, peptide conjugation capacity, organ reserve, and other genetic and non genetic factors determines their toxic tolerance. Every individual is different. Total avoidance and elimination should be the practice.

A mild detoxification regimen that I have used on individuals who are too sick to treat aggressively is to recommend taking Chlorella Pyrenoidosa at bedtime. Chlorella Pyrenoidosa is a sea alga which binds organic pollutants and heavy metals and limits their reabsorption. This works well in most patients without interfering with their other treatment regimens.

Chlorella is often given with cilantro also known as coriander or Chinese parsley, and/or with spirulina, an intense super food bacterium often misidentified as blue-green algae. These agents increase the elimination of heavy metals and other toxins and provide a source of amino acids and energy. Amino acids are necessary for peptide conjugation in second-phase detoxification.

Chlorella contains a high amount of chlorophyll and has been used as an adjunct during radiation treatment. The chlorophyll protects against ultraviolet radiation. The tough, fibrous material in the outer shell binds the toxins and metals and carries them out of the body. This super food is comprised of 60% protein, 18 amino acids including all of the essential amino acids required by the human body, and various vitamins and minerals. Chlorella Growth Factor, CGF, a phytonutrient containing RNA and DNA, provides the building blocks for the repair of our genetic material.

Spirulina is similar to Chlorella in nutrient value but lacks the cell wall found in plants. The protein content is similar. Additionally, it provides omega-3 fatty acids and antioxidants which provide protective value to the regimen.

Toxins, particularly heavy metals through the production of free radicals and their ionizing charges, can increase clotting and provoke inflammation. Additionally, because store-bought foods contain reduced amounts of omega-3 fatty acids, these problems are often aggravated by our low omega-3 diets. Omega-3 fatty acid supplementation or consuming foods high in omega-3 to reduce inflammation can be very beneficial for most people.

An excellent vegetable source for omega-3 is Chia (Salvia hispanica), a plant that is native to Mexico. The 2 mm seed is frequently served at salad bars as sprouts. The Chia pet is a common find in novelty stores.

According to Dr. Vuksans' findings on Salba-brand Chia, appearing in the article "Seeds of Wellness: Return of a Supergrain" in *The Saturday Evening Post* (November 15, 2007), Chia contains eight times the amount of omega-3 as salmon, and is a good source for B vitamins, folic acid, amino acids, vitamin C, calcium, and iron.

Chia flour or meal can be used for baking, and has negligible gluten. Chia meal also makes a good thickener for soups and other foods and can add to the nutritional value of meatloaf, burgers, or meat balls by mixing it in with the meat. The meal can be added to all sorts of foods to increase their nutritional value. This is especially important for picky eaters and the elderly. The seeds should be ground prior to ingestion to maximize nutrient acquisition as they can pass whole in some individuals due to their tough outer shell.

The primary fatty acids in chia are alpha-linolenic acid (ALA) and gamma-linolenic acid (GLA). The body converts α-linolenic acid into the longer chain fatty acids Eicosapentaenoic acid (EPA) and docosahexaenoic acid DHA which are abundant in fish. ALA is the parent fatty acid. Some health advocates claim the ALA/GLA combination provides better membrane benefits for improved cellular oxygenation than EPA / DHA or fish oils.

Since Chia seeds absorb water when left to stand, some folks consume the whole seed (2 heaping table-spoons) in a glass of water or juice 30 minutes before mealtime to create a sensation of fullness so as to suppress their appetite.

The seeds are considered a perfect food. One can survive on Chia and water for long periods of time, and they were used by the Aztec Indians for such purposes on long trips. Stored dry, the seeds can retain their nutritional value for up to five years. This makes it an excellent food for times of scarcity. Since Chia grows easily, it is an excellent plant for ending world hunger and malnutrition. Many in South Texas and Mexico have it growing wild in their yards.

Oxidation, the free radical consumption of electrons creating damaging by products, is the major mechanism of damage caused by toxins, radiation, inflamation, stress, and aging. Oxygenation can contribute electrons to the system and is not the same as oxidation. Free radicals of oxygen, however, can induce oxidation.

Foods and nutritional supplements that target oxidation, such as antioxidants, should be a daily routine. Avoiding oxidative agents, toxins, tobacco, and unnecesary drugs can help reduce a person's oxidative burden. The excessive intake of calories can also add to a person's oxidative stress and should influence your choice of foods and the quantity that you consume.

Consuming foods that increase a person's ability to rid their body of toxic agents is very important. Proteins, which provide amino acids for peptide conjugation, a phase-two detoxification pathway, are very important.

Glutathione is one of the more important amino acids for detoxification. A problem in many disease states is low glutathione levels. The list of diseases recognized as having low glutathione levels is quite long. Such individuals require more glutathione enriching foods.

Glutathione does not cross the cell membrane. The cell must manufacture its own glutathione from its precursor amino acids, cystine, glycine, and glutamate. Circulating glutathione assist in cell immunity by attaching to the microbe and attracting immune cells which engulf and destroy the microbe.

Asparagus, broccoli, avocado, and spinach increase glutathione levels. Eggs, unprocessed meats, and garlic are good sources of high sulphur-containing amino acids which help raise glutathione levels.

Raw whole foods are prefered since they provide more complete nutrition than most supplements. Such foods provide the various vitalnutrients needed for metabolic reactions, thus are a more wholistic method of helping body processes.

Individuals who do not consume sufficient vegetables are at a disadvantage. They can suffer nutritional deficiencies, impairing the body's detoxification. This can cause toxins to accumulate since the toxins cannot be mobilized and removed from the body.

Juicing is an acceptable substitute and prefered in individuals who cannot chew adequately. Another way is to take natural concentrated encapsulated fruits and vegetables. Individuals who do not consume the 7 or more daily servings of fruits and vegetables should consider one of these alternatives. Encapsulated fruits and vegetables and related information can be found on the web at **www. drcaquias4juiceplus.com**

For supplements, I generally recommend products by Pure Encapsulation, (1) B6 complex with methyl B12 and methyl folate, taken daily, (2) Digestive Enzymes Ultra, taken before meals, (3) 20 billion of mixed probiotics with lactobacillus and bifidobacterium, taken after a meal, and (4) two to four Ultra Nutients taken daily. The methyl B12 and methyl folate support methylation, a major detoxification pathway impaired in many individuals. Supplementating with B12 and folic acid and B6 on a regular basis has been shown to help prevent brain atrophy and alzheimers. These products can be obtained on the web at **purecap-spro.com/drcaquias**.

In summary, the recommendations are: high nutrition low caloric foods, adequate exercise and sleep, good hydration and bowel function, some form of detoxification, and supplemention with nutrients that support membrane and mitochondria function, detoxification, and reduce oxidative stress.

Finally, good health requires an optimistic attitude. The scriptures provide us with the assurance that, regardless of how bad things seem, the finality is controlled by the one who cannot fail us. We can trust in His reward and all that He has promised us.

Remember when trials come, as long as you trust and are in obedience, He will guide you through it. Regardless of the end result – even onto death – He will take care of you, *"... do not fear those who kill the body but cannot kill the soul. But rather fear Him who is able to destroy both soul and body in hell." (Matthew 10:28 NKJV)* *

With this assurance, we can face the challenges of life unafraid for He is always with us. The trials and tribulations are the chisels and hammers sculpturing us into the masterpieces we are to become. His Word advises us: *"My son, give attention to my words; Incline your ear to my sayings. Do not let them depart from your eyes; Keep them in the midst of your heart; For they are life to those who find them, And health to all their flesh. Keep your heart with all diligence, For out of it spring the issues of life." (Proverbs 4:20–23 NKJV)* *

Chapter 20

1. Disciplining oneself to eat right takes as much fortitude and willpower as keeping a _____; the more or longer you do it, the easier it is.

2. When exercising for health, never work yourself to the point of pain or _____, as this is your body warning you that you are exceeding the body's limit.

3. Give yourself adequate time between exercises for your body to _____, and remember that rest is as important as exercise.

4. Exercise to counter the effects of gravity on your body when possible with spinal _____ exercises, such as pull-ups or pulling weights down rather than lifting heavy objects that compress your spine.

5. Distributing your water intake over the entire day is more beneficial than drinking large amounts at once because it is better _____ and not rapidly eliminated by the body.

6. Electrical pollutants which have _____ a millionfold over the past 10 years likewise augment the toxic effects of biological toxins.

Answers: fast, exhaustion, recuperate, stretching, distributed, increased

Old Testament Messianic Prophesies and their New Testament Fulfillment

•

Messiah would come by the seed of a Woman, a virgen:

Old Testament

"And I will put enmity between you and the woman, And between your seed and her Seed; ...." (Genesis 3:15 NKJV)*

"Therefore the Lord Himself will give you a sign: Behold, the virgin shall conceive and bear a Son, and shall call His name Immanuel (God is with us)." (Isaiah 7:14 NKJV)*

New Testament

"And the angel answered and said to her, "The Holy Spirit will come upon you, and the power of the Highest will overshadow you; therefore, also, that Holy One who is to be born will be called the Son of God." (Luke 1:35 NKJV)*

"Now the birth of Jesus Christ was as follows: After His mother Mary was betrothed to Joseph, before they came together, she was found with child of the Holy Spirit." (Matthew 1:18 NKJV)*

•

Messiah would strike Satan at the head:

Old Testament

"And I will put enmity between you and the woman, And between your seed and her Seed; He shall bruise your head, And you shall bruise His heel." (Genesis 3:15 NKJV)*

New Testament

"Inasmuch then as the children have partaken of flesh and blood, He Himself likewise shared in the same, that through death He might

destroy him who had the power of death, that is, the devil," (Hebrews 2:14 NKJV)*

•

Messiah a priest and King after Melchizedek, the King of peace (Salem), foreshadow of the last supper:

Old Testament
"Then Melchizedek king of Salem brought out bread and wine; he was the priest of God Most High. And he blessed him..." (Genesis 14:18 NKJV)*

New Testament
"...where the forerunner has entered for us, even Jesus, having become High Priest forever according to the order of Melchizedek." (Hebrews 6:20 NKJV)*

•

Messiah to come from the seed of Isaac:

Old Testament
"Then God said: "No, Sarah your wife shall bear you a son, and you shall call his name Isaac; I will establish My covenant with him for an everlasting covenant, and with his descendants after him." (Genesis 17:19 NKJV)*

New Testament
"Now to Abraham and his Seed were the promises made. He does not say, "And to seeds," as of many, but as of one, "And to your Seed,"who is Christ." (Galatians 3:16 NKJV)*

•

Messiah the son of God:

Old Testament
"Who has ascended into heaven, or descended? Who has gathered the wind in His fists? Who has bound the waters in a garment? Who has

232

established all the ends of the earth? What is His name, and what is His Son's name, If you know?" (Proverbs 30:4 NKJV)*

"Also I will make him My firstborn, The highest of the kings of the earth. My mercy I will keep for him forever, And My covenant shall stand firm with him. His seed (His true followers) also I will make to endure forever, And his throne as the days of heaven." (Psalm 89:27-29NKJV)*

New Testament
"No one has ascended to heaven but He who came down from heaven, that is, the Son of Man who is in heaven." (John 3:13 NKJV)*

"...concerning His Son Jesus Christ our Lord, who was born of the seed of David according to the flesh, and declared to be the Son of God with power according to the Spirit of holiness, by the resurrection from the dead. Through Him we have received grace and apostleship for obedience to the faith among all nations for His name," (Romans 1:3-5 NKJV)*

"For He received from God the Father honor and glory when such a voice came to Him from the Excellent Glory: "This is My beloved Son, in whom I am well pleased." And we heard this voice which came from heaven when we were with Him on the holy mountain." (2 Peter 1:17,18 NKJV)*

"When He had been baptized, Jesus came up immediately from the water; and behold, the heavens were opened to Him, and He saw the Spirit of God descending like a dove and alighting upon Him. And suddenly a voice came from heaven, saying, "This is My beloved Son, in whom I am well pleased." (Matthew 3:16,17 NKJV)*

•

God to provide the lamb:

Old Testament
"And Abraham said, "My son, God will provide for Himself the lamb for a burnt offering." So the two of them went together." (Genesis 22:8 NKJV)*

New Testament
"The next day John saw Jesus coming toward him, and said, "Behold! The Lamb of God who takes away the sin of the world!" (John 1:29 NKJV)*

•

Messiah must be perfect, a lamb without blemish:

Old Testament
"Your lamb shall be without blemish, a male of the first year. You may take it from the sheep or from the goats." (Exodus 12:5 NKJV)*

New Testament
"but with the precious blood of Christ, as of a lamb without blemish and without spot." (1 Peter 1:19 NKJV)*

•

Not a bone of the lamb (Messiah) to be broken:

Old Testament
"In one house it shall be eaten; you shall not carry any of the flesh outside the house, nor shall you break one of its bones." (Exodus 12:46 NKJV)*

"They shall leave none of it until morning, nor break one of its bones. According to all the ordinances of the Passover they shall keep it. " (Numbers 9:12 NKJV)*

New Testament
"Therefore, because it was the Preparation Day, that the bodies should not remain on the cross on the Sabbath (for that Sabbath was a high day), the Jews asked Pilate that their legs might be broken, and that they might be taken away. Then the soldiers came and broke the legs of the first and of the other who was crucified with Him. But when they came to Jesus and saw that He was already dead, they did not break His legs." (John 19:31-33 NKJV)*

•

The first born to be consecrated:

Old Testament

"Then the LORD spoke to Moses, saying, "Consecrate to Me all the firstborn, whatever opens the womb among the children of Israel, both of man and beast; it is Mine." (Exodus 13:2 NKJV)*

New Testament

"And she brought forth her firstborn Son, and wrapped Him in swaddling cloths, and laid Him in a manger, because there was no room for them in the inn." (Luke 2:7 NKJV)*

•

God to be their Yahshua (salvation):

Old Testament

"The LORD is my strength and song, And He has become my salvation; He is my God, and I will praise Him; My father's God, and I will exalt Him." (Exodus 15:2 NKJV)*

"Behold, God is my salvation, I will trust and not be afraid; ' For YAH, the LORD, is my strength and song; He also has become my salvation." (Isaiah 12:2 NKJV)*

New Testament

"Jesus said to him, "I am the way, the truth, and the life. No one comes to the Father except through Me." (John 14:6 NKJV)*

"And she will bring forth a Son, and you shall call His name Jesus (Yashua), for He will save His people from their sins." (Matthew 1:21 NKJV)*

•

A God glorious in holiness and doing wonders:

Old Testament

"Who is like You, O LORD, among the gods? Who is like You, glorious in holiness, Fearful in praises, doing wonders?" (Exodus 15:11 NKJV)*

"looking for the blessed hope and glorious appearing of our great God and Savior Jesus Christ," (Titus 2:13 NKJV)*

•

The blood that makes atonement must be taken outside the gate:

Old Testament
"The bull for the sin offering and the goat for the sin offering, whose blood was brought in to make atonement in the Holy Place, shall be carried outside the camp. And they shall burn in the fire their skins, their flesh, and their offal." (Leviticus 16:27 NKJV)*

New Testament
"For the bodies of those animals, whose blood is brought into the sanctuary by the high priest for sin, are burned outside the camp. Therefore Jesus also, that He might sanctify the people with His own blood, suffered outside the gate." (Hebrew 13:11,12 NKJV)*

•

Like the serpent on a pole Messiah must be lifted up for healing:

Old Testament
"So Moses made a bronze serpent, and put it on a pole; and so it was, if a serpent had bitten anyone, when he looked at the bronze serpent, he lived." (Numbers 21:9)*

New Testament
"And as Moses lifted up the serpent in the wilderness, even so must the Son of Man be lifted up, that whoever believes in Him should not perish but have eternal life." (John 3:14,15 NKJV)*

•

God to bring Messiah out of Egypt:

Old Testament
"God brings him out of Egypt; He has strength like a wild ox; He shall consume the nations, his enemies; He shall break their bones And pierce them with his arrows." (Numbers 24:8 NKJV)*

"When Israel was a child, I loved him And out of Egypt I called My son." (Hosea 11:1 NKJV)*

New Testament
"When he arose, he took the young Child and His mother by night and departed for Egypt, and was there until the death of Herod, that it might be fulfilled which was spoken by the Lord through the prophet, saying, "Out of Egypt I called My Son." (Matthew 2:14,15 NKJV)*

●

Messiah shall come as a prophet like Moses:

Old Testament
"The LORD your God will raise up for you a Prophet like me from your midst, from your brethren. Him you shall hear," (Deuteronomy 18:15 NKJV)*

"I will raise up for them a Prophet like you from among their brethren, and will put My words in His mouth, and He shall speak to them all that I command Him." (Deuteronomy 18:18 NKJV)*

And it shall be that whoever will not hear My words, which He speaks in My name, I will require it of him." (Deuteronomy 18:18 NKJV)*

New Testament
"He will glorify Me, for He will take of what is Mine and declare it to you." (John 16:14 NKJV)*

●

237

Messiah shall not hang on the tree overnight, cursed is he that hangs from the tree:

Old Testament
"his body shall not remain overnight on the tree, but you shall surely bury him that day, so that you do not defile the land which the LORD your God is giving you as an inheritance; for he who is hanged is accursed of God." (Deuteronomy 21:23 NKJV)*

New Testament
"For as many as are of the works of the law are under the curse; for it is written, "Cursed is everyone who does not continue in all things which are written in the book of the law, to do them." But that no one is justified by the law in the sight of God is evident, for "the just shall live by faith." Yet the law is not of faith, but "the man who does them shall live by them." Christ has redeemed us from the curse of the law, having become a curse for us (for it is written, "Cursed is everyone who hangs on a tree")," (Galatians 3:10-13 NKJV)*

"Therefore, because it was the Preparation Day, that the bodies should not remain on the cross on the Sabbath (for that Sabbath was a high day), the Jews asked Pilate that their legs might be broken, and that they might be taken away. Then the soldiers came and broke the legs of the first and of the other who was crucified with Him. But when they came to Jesus and saw that He was already dead, they did not break His legs. But one of the soldiers pierced His side with a spear, and immediately blood and water came out" (John 19:31-34 NKJV)*

•

Messiah shall come from the seed of King David:

Old Testament
"When your days (David) are fulfilled and you rest with your fathers, I will set up your seed after you, who will come from your body, and I will establish his kingdom."(2 Samuel 7:12 NKJV)*

New Testament
"The book of the genealogy of Jesus Christ, the Son of David, the Son of Abraham:" (Matthew 1:1 NKJV)* (Joseph and Mary were both of the lineage of David)

•

Messiah is the rock:

Old Testament
"The Spirit of the LORD spoke by me, And His word was on my tongue. The God of Israel said, The Rock of Israel spoke to me:" (2 Samuel 23:2-3 NKJV08)*

"The LORD is my rock and my fortress and my deliverer; My God, my strength, in whom I will trust; My shield and the horn of my salvation, my stronghold." (Psalm 18:2 NKJV)*

New Testment
"...and all drank the same spiritual drink. For they drank of that spiritual Rock that followed them, and that Rock was Christ." (1 Corinthians 10:4 NKJV)*

•

Messiah is the light of the morning:

Old Testament
"And he shall be like the light of the morning when the sun rises, A morning without clouds, Like the tender grass springing out of the earth, By clear shining after rain." (2 Samuel 23:4 NKJV)*

New Testament
"I, Jesus, have sent My angel to testify to you these things in the churches. I am the Root and the Offspring of David, the Bright and Morning Star." (Revelation 22:16 NKJV)*

•

Messiah's throne shall be forever:

Old Testament
"He shall build Me a house, and I will establish his throne forever. I will be his Father, and he shall be My son; and I will not take My mercy away from him, as I took it from him who was before you." (1 Chronicles 17:12 NKJV)*

New Testament
"He will be great, and will be called the Son of the Highest; and the Lord God will give Him the throne of His father David. And He will reign over the house of Jacob forever, and of His kingdom there will be no end." (Luke 1:32,33 NKJV)*

•

God to be Messiah's father:

Old Testament
"He shall build Me a house, and I will establish his throne forever. I will be his Father, and he shall be My son; and I will not take My mercy away from him, as I took it from him who was before you." (1 Chronicles 17:12 NKJV)*

New Testament
"For to which of the angels did He ever say: "You are My Son,Today I have begotten You"? And again: "I will be to Him a Father, And He shall be to Me a Son"? (Hebrews 1:5 NKJV)

•

Messiah resurrected to dispense life and judgment:

Old Testament
"For I know that my Redeemer lives, And He shall stand at last on the earth; And after my skin is destroyed, this I know, That in my flesh I shall see God, Whom I shall see for myself, And my eyes shall behold, and not another. How my heart yearns within me! If you should say, 'How shall we persecute him?'Since the root of the matter is found in me, Be afraid

of the sword for yourselves; For wrath brings the punishment of the sword, That you may know there is a judgment." (Job 19:25-29 NKJV)*

New Testament

"Most assuredly, I say to you, he who hears My word and believes in Him who sent Me has everlasting life, and shall not come into judgment, but has passed from death into life. Most assuredly, I say to you, the hour is coming, and now is, when the dead will hear the voice of the Son of God; and those who hear will live. For as the Father has life in Himself, so He has granted the Son to have life in Himself, and has given Him authority to execute judgment also, because He is the Son of Man. Do not marvel at this; for the hour is coming in which all who are in the graves will hear His voice and come forth—those who have done good, to the resurrection of life, and those who have done evil, to the resurrection of condemnation." (John 5:24-29 NKJV)*

"Now therefore, be wise, O kings; Be instructed, you judges of the earth. Serve the LORD with fear, And rejoice with trembling. Kiss the Son, lest He be angry, And you perish in the way," (Psalm 2:10-12 NKJV)*

•

Messiah shall not to see corruption:

Old Testament

"For You will not leave my soul in Sheol, Nor will You allow Your Holy One to see corruption." (Psalm 16:10 NKJV)*

New Testament

"....He would raise up the Christ to sit on his throne, he, foreseeing this, spoke concerning the resurrection of the Christ, that His soul was not left in Hades, nor did His flesh see corruption. This Jesus God has raised up, of which we are all witnesses. Therefore being exalted to the right hand of God, and having received from the Father the promise of the Holy Spirit, He poured out this which you now see and hear. "For David did not ascend into the heavens, but he says himself: The LORD said to my Lord, " Sit at My right hand,Till I make Your enemies Your footstool." (Acts 2;30-35 NKJV)*

•

241

Messiah to be forsaken for the sins of others:

Old Testament

"My God, My God, why have You forsaken Me? Why are You so far from helping Me, And from the words of My groaning?" (Psalm 22:1 NKJV)*

New Testament

"For He made Him who knew no sin to be sin for us, that we might become the righteousness of God in Him." (2 Corinthians 5:21 NKJV)*

•

Messiah crucified:

Old Testament

"Many bulls have surrounded Me; Strong bulls of Bashan have encircled Me. They gape at Me with their mouths, Like a raging and roaring lion. I am poured out like water, And all My bones are out of joint; My heart is like wax; It has melted within Me. My strength is dried up like a potsherd, And My tongue clings to My jaws; You have brought Me to the dust of death. For dogs have surrounded Me; The congregation of the wicked has enclosed Me. They pierced My hands and My feet; I can count all My bones. They look and stare at Me. They divide My garments among them, And for My clothing they cast lots." (Psalm 22:12-18 NKJV)*

"He is despised and rejected by men, A Man of sorrows and acquainted with grief. And we hid, as it were, our faces from Him; He was despised, and we did not esteem Him. Surely He has borne our griefs And carried our sorrows; Yet we esteemed Him stricken, Smitten by God, and afflicted. But He was wounded for our transgressions. He was bruised for our iniquities; The chastisement for our peace was upon Him, And by His stripes we are healed. All we like sheep have gone astray; We have turned, every one, to his own way; And the LORD has laid on Him the iniquity of us all. He was oppressed and He was afflicted, Yet He opened not His mouth; He was led as a lamb to the slaughter, And as a sheep before its shearers is silent, So He opened not His mouth. He was taken from prison and from judgment, And who will declare His genera-tion. For He was cut off from the land of the living; For the transgressions of My people He was stricken. And they made His grave with the wicked But with the rich at His death, Because He had done no

violence, Nor was any deceit in His mouth. Yet it pleased the LORD to bruise Him; He has put Him to grief. When You make His soul an offering for sin, He shall see His seed, He shall prolong His days, And the pleasure of the LORD shall prosper in His hand. He shall see the labor of His soul, and be satisfied. By His knowledge My righteous Servant shall justify many, For He shall bear their iniquities." (Isaiah 53:3-11 NKJV)*

New Testament
"Then the soldiers of the governor took Jesus into the Praetorium and gathered the whole garrison around Him. And they stripped Him and put a scarlet robe on Him. When they had twisted a crown of thorns, they put it on His head, and a reed in His right hand. And they bowed the knee before Him and mocked Him, saying, "Hail, King of the Jews!" Then they spat on Him, and took the reed and struck Him on the head. And when they had mocked Him, they took the robe off Him, put His own clothes on Him, and led Him away to be crucified. Now as they came out, they found a man of Cyrene, Simon by name. Him they compelled to bear His cross. And when they had come to a place called Golgotha, that is to say, Place of a Skull, they gave Him sour wine mingled with gall to drink. But when He had tasted it, He would not drink. Then they crucified Him, and divided His garments, casting lots, that it might be fulfilled which was spoken by the prophet: "They divided My garments among them, And for My clothing they cast lots." Sitting down, they kept watch over Him there. And they put up over His head the accusation written against Him: THIS IS JESUS THE KING OF THE JEWS." (Matthew:27-36 NKJV)*

•

Messiah betrayed by a friend who ate bread with Him:

Old Testament
"Even my own familiar friend in whom I trusted, Who ate my bread, Has lifted up his heel against me." (Psalm 41:9 NKJV)*

New Testament
"I do not speak concerning all of you. I know whom I have chosen; but that the Scripture may be fulfilled, 'He who eats bread with Me has lifted up his heel against Me.' (John 13:18 NKJV)*

•

Messiah shall dispense grace from His lips:

Old Testament
"You are fairer than the sons of men; Grace is poured upon Your lips; Therefore God has blessed You forever." (Psalm 45:2 NKJV)*

New Testament
"So all bore witness to Him, and marveled at the gracious words which proceeded out of His mouth. And they said, "Is this not Joseph's son?" (Luke 4:22 NKJV)*

•

Messiah owner of the title of God, Elohim:

Old Testament
"Your throne, O God, is forever and ever; A scepter of righteousness is the scepter of Your kingdom. You love righteousness and hate wickedness; Therefore God, Your God, has anointed You With the oil of gladness more than Your companions." (Psalm 45:6-7 NKJV)*

"For unto us a Child is born, Unto us a Son is given; And the government will be upon His shoulder. And His name will be called Wonderful, Counselor, Mighty God, Everlasting Father, Prince of Peace." (Isaiah 9:6 NKJV)*

New Testament
"But to the Son He says:" Your throne, O God, is forever and ever; A scepter of righteousness is the scepter of Your kingdom." (Hebrews 1:8 NKJV)*

"In the beginning was the Word, and the Word was with God, and the Word was God. He was in the beginning with God. All things were made through Him, and without Him nothing was made that was made. In Him was life, and the life was the light of men. And the light shines in the darkness, and the darkness did not comprehend it." (John 1:1-5 NKJV)*

•

Kings shall visit Messiah and bring presents:

Old Testament
"The kings of Tarshish and of the isles Will bring presents; The kings of Sheba and Seba Will offer gifts. Yes, all kings shall fall down before Him; All nations shall serve Him." (Psalm 72:10 NKJV)*

New Testament
"Now after Jesus was born in Bethlehem of Judea in the days of Herod the king, behold, wise men from the East came to Jerusalem, saying, "Where is He who has been born King of the Jews? For we have seen His star in the East and have come to worship Him." (Matthew 2:1-2 NKJV)*

When they saw the star, they rejoiced with exceedingly great joy. And when they had come into the house, they saw the young Child with Mary His mother, and fell down and worshiped Him. And when they had opened their treasures, they presented gifts to Him: gold, frankincense, and myrrh. Then, being divinely warned in a dream that they should not return to Herod, they departed for their own country another way." (Matthew 2:10-12 NKJV)*

•

Messiah will teach in parables:

Old Testament
"Give ear, O my people, to my law; incline your ears to the words of my mouth I will open my mouth in a parable; I will utter dark sayings of old," (Psalm 78:1-2 NKJV)*

New Testament
"All these things Jesus spoke to the multitude in parables; and without a parable He did not speak to them, that it might be fulfilled which was spoken by the prophet, saying: " I will open My Mouth in parables; I will utter things kept secret from the foundation of the world." (Matthew 13:34-35 NKJV)*

•

Messiah shall call God "Father":

Old Testament
"He shall cry to Me, 'You are my Father, My God, and the rock of my salvation.'" (Psalm 89:26 NKJV)*

New Testament
"All things have been delivered to Me by My Father, and no one knows the Son except the Father. Nor does anyone know the Father except the Son, and the one to whom the Son wills to reveal Him." (Matthew 11:27 NKJV)*

•

God's firstborn Yahshua and His seed (followers) to endure forever:

Old Testament
"Also I will make him My firstborn, The highest of the kings of the earth. My mercy I will keep for him forever, And My covenant shall stand firm with him. His seed (His followers) also I will make to endure forever, And his throne as the days of heaven." (Psalm 89:27-29NKJV)*

"His seed shall endure forever, And his throne as the sun before Me; It shall be established forever like the moon, Even like the faithful witness in the sky." Selah" (Psalm 89:36,37 NKJV)*

New Testament
"He will be great, and will be called the Son of the Highest; and the Lord God will give Him the throne of His father David. And He will reign over the house of Jacob forever, and of His kingdom there will be no end." (Luke 1:32-33 NKJV)*

"For God so loved the world that He gave His only begotten Son, that whoever believes in Him should not perish but have everlasting life. For God did not send His Son into the world to condemn the world, but that the world through Him might be saved. "He who believes in Him is not condemned; but he who does not believe is condemned already, because he has not believed in the name of the only begotten Son of God." (John 3:16-18 NKJV)*

•

Messiah is from everlasting:

Old Testament

Before the mountains were brought forth, Or ever You had formed the earth and the world, Even from everlasting to everlasting, You are God." (Psalm 90:2)

"But you, Bethlehem Ephrathah, Though you are little among the thousands of Judah, Yet out of you shall come forth to Me The One to be Ruler in Israel, Whose goings forth are from of old, From everlasting." (Micah 5:2 NKJV)*

"The LORD possessed me at the beginning of His way, Before His works of old. I have been established from everlasting, From the beginning, before there was ever an earth."(Proverbs 8:22-23 NKJV)*

New Testament

"In the beginning was the Word, and the Word was with God, and the Word was God."(John 1:1 NKJV)*

Jesus said to them, "Most assuredly, I say to you, before Abraham was, I AM."(John 8:58 NKJV)*

•

Messiah a target of the devil:

Old Testament

For He shall give His angels charge over you, To keep you in all your ways.In their hands they shall bear you up, Lest you dash your foot against a stone." (Psalm 91:11,12 NKJV)*

New Testament

Then he (the devil) brought Him to Jerusalem, set Him on the pinnacle of the temple, and said to Him, "If You are the Son of God, throw Yourself down from here. For it is written: 'He shall give His angels charge over you, To keep you' and,' In their hands they shall bear you up, Lest you dash your foot against a stone.'"And Jesus answered and said to him, "It

247

has been said, 'You shall not tempt the LORD your God.'"Now when the devil had ended every temptation, he departed from Him until an opportune time." (Luke 4:9-13 NKJV)*

•

Only God is to be worshipped:

Old Testament

*Let all be put to shame who serve carved images, Who boast of idols. Worship Him, all you gods. Zion hears and is glad, And the daughters of Judah rejoice Because of Your judgments, O LORD. For You, LORD, are most high above all the earth; You are exalted far above all gods. You who love the LORD, hate evil! He preserves the souls of His saints; He delivers them out of the hand of the wicked (Psalm 97: 7-10 NKJV)**

*"You shall not make for yourself a carved image—any likeness of anything that is in heaven above, or that is in the earth beneath, or that is in the water under the earth; you shall not bow down to them nor serve them. For I, the LORD your God, am a jealous God, visiting the iniquity of the fathers upon the children to the third and fourth generations of those who hate Me, (Exodus 20:4-5 NKJV)**

New Testament

*"Then Jesus said to him, "Away with you, Satan! For it is written, 'You shall worship the LORD your God, and Him only you shall serve " (Matthew 4:10 NKJV)**

*"As Peter was coming in, Cornelius met him and fell down at his feet and worshiped him. But Peter lifted him up, saying, "Stand up; I myself am also a man." (Acts 10:25-26 NKJV)**

*"Beware lest anyone cheat you through philosophy and empty deceit, according to the tradition of men, according to the basic principles of the world, and not according to Christ. For in Him dwells all the fullness of the Godhead bodily; and you are complete in Him, who is the head of all principality and power." (Colossians 2:8-10 NKJV)**

"Let no one cheat you of your reward, taking delight in false humility and worship of angels, intruding into those things which he has not seen,

vainly puffed up by his fleshly mind, and not holding fast to the Head (which is Christ), from whom all the body, nourished and knit together by joints and ligaments, grows with the increase that is from God." (Colossians 2:18,19 NKJV)*

"Then he said to me, "Write: 'Blessed are those who are called to the marriage supper of the Lamb!'" And he said to me, "These are the true sayings of God." And I fell at his feet to worship him. But he said to me, "See that you do not do that! I am your fellow servant, and of your brethren who have the testimony of Jesus. Worship God! For the testimony of Jesus is the spirit of prophecy." (Revelation 19:9,10 NKJV)*

"He who overcomes shall inherit all things, and I will be his God and he shall be My son. But the cowardly, unbelieving, abominable, murderers, sexually immoral, sorcerers, idolaters, and all liars shall have their part in the lake which burns with fire and brimstone, which is the second death."(Revelation 21:7,8 NKJV)*

•

The rejected stone (Yahshua) becomes the chief corner stone:

Old Testament
"The stone which the builders rejected Has become the chief cornerstone. This was the LORD's doing; It is marvelous in our eyes." (Psalm 18:22,23 NKJV)*

"Therefore thus says the Lord GOD: " Behold, I lay in Zion a stone for a foundation, A tried stone, a precious cornerstone, a sure foundation; Whoever believes will not act hastily." (Isaiah 28:16 NKJV)*

New Testament
"Jesus said to them, "Have you never read in the Scriptures: The stone which the builders rejected Has become the chief cornerstoneThis was the LORD's doing, And it is marvelous in our eyes'? "Therefore I say to you, the kingdom of God will be taken from you and given to a nation bearing the fruits of it. And whoever falls on this stone will be broken; but on whomever it falls, it will grind him to powder." (Matthew 21:42,43 NKJV)*

•

Messiah shall come while the Temple (House of the Lord) is standing:

Old Testament

"Blessed is he who comes in the name of the LORD! We have blessed you from the house of the LORD." (Psalm 18:26 NKJV)*

New Testament

So the disciples went and did as Jesus commanded them. They brought the donkey and the colt, laid their clothes on them, and set Him on them. And a very great multitude spread their clothes on the road; others cut down branches from the trees and spread them on the road. Then the multitudes who went before and those who followed cried out, saying: "Hosanna to the Son of David! Blessed is He who comes in the name of the LORD!' Hosanna in the highest!" And when He had come into Jerusalem, all the city was moved, saying, "Who is this?" So the multitudes said, "This is Jesus, the prophet from Nazareth of Galilee." (Matthew 21:6-11 NKJV)*

•

Messiah Yahshua's ministry in Jerusalem:

Old Testament

"The LORD builds up Jerusalem; He gathers together the outcasts of Israel. He heals the brokenhearted And binds up their wounds. He counts the number of the stars; He calls them all by name. Great is our Lord, and mighty in power; His understanding is infinite. The LORD lifts up the humble; He casts the wicked down to the ground." (Psalm 147:2-6 NKJV)*

New Testament

So He came to Nazareth, where He had been brought up. And as His custom was, He went into the synagogue on the Sabbath day, and stood up to read. And He was handed the book of the prophet Isaiah. And when He had opened the book, He found the place where it was written: "The Spirit of the LORD is upon Me,Because He has anointed Me To preach the gospel to the poor; He has sent Me to heal the broken- hearted, To proclaim liberty to the captives And recovery of sight to the blind, To set at liberty those who are oppressed;To proclaim the

acceptable year of the LORD." Then He closed the book, and gave it back to the attendant and sat down. And the eyes of all who were in the synagogue were fixed on Him. And He began to say to them, "Today this Scripture is fulfilled in your hearing." (Luke 4:16-21 NKJV)*
Now the Passover of the Jews was at hand, and Jesus went up to Jerusalem. And He found in the temple those who sold oxen and sheep and doves, and the money changers doing business. When He had made a whip of cords, He drove them all out of the temple, with the sheep and the oxen, and poured out the changers' money and overturned the tables. And He said to those who sold doves, "Take these things away! Do not make My Father's house a house of merchandise!" Then His disciples remembered that it was written, "Zeal for Your house has eaten Me up." (John 2:13-17 NKJV)*

•

Yahshua's ministry to begin in Galilee:

Old Testament
"Nevertheless the gloom will not be upon her who is distressed, As when at first He lightly esteemed The land of Zebulun and the land of Naphtali, And afterward more heavily oppressed her, By the way of the sea, beyond the Jordan, In Galilee of the Gentiles. The people who walked in darkness Have seen a great light; Those who dwelt in the land of the shadow of death, Upon them a light has shined. " (Isaiah 9:1,2 NKJV)*

New Testament
"Now when Jesus heard that John had been put in prison, He departed to Galilee. And leaving Nazareth, He came and dwelt in Capernaum, which is by the sea, in the regions of Zebulun and Naphtali, that it might be fulfilled which was spoken by Isaiah the prophet, saying:" The land of Zebulun and the land of Naphtali, By the way of the sea, beyond the Jordan, Galilee of the Gentiles: The people who sat in darkness have seen a great light, And upon those who sat in the region and shadow of death Light has dawned." From that time Jesus began to preach and to say, "Repent, for the kingdom of heaven is at hand."(Matthew 4:12-17 NKJV)*

•

251

God gives us His son for an everlasting government:

Old Testament
"For unto us a Child is born, Unto us a Son is given; And the government will be upon His shoulder. And His name will be called Wonderful, Counselor, Mighty God, Everlasting Father, Prince of Peace. Of the increase of His government and peace There will be no end, Upon the throne of David and over His kingdom, To order it and establish it with judgment and justice From that time forward, even forever. The zeal of the Lord of hosts will perform this. (Isaiah 9:6,7 NKJV)*

New Testament
"And behold, you will conceive in your womb and bring forth a Son, and shall call His name JESUS. He will be great, and will be called the Son of the Highest; and the Lord God will give Him the throne of His father David. And He will reign over the house of Jacob forever, and of His kingdom there will be no end."(Luke 1:31-33 NKJV)*

"And without controversy great is the mystery of godliness: God was manifested in the flesh, Justified in the Spirit, Seen by angels, Preached among the Gentiles, Believed on in the world, Received up in glory." (1 Timothy 3:16 NKJV)*

"When He had come to His own country, He taught them in their synagogue, so that they were astonished and said, "Where did this Man get this wisdom and these mighty works? (Matthew 13:54 NKJV)*

"Then He began to rebuke the cities in which most of His mighty works had been done, because they did not repent: "Woe to you, Chorazin! Woe to you, Bethsaida! For if the mighty works which were done in you had been done in Tyre and Sidon, they would have repented long ago in sackcloth and ashes. But I say to you, it will be more tolerable for Tyre and Sidon in the day of judgment than for you. And you, Capernaum, who are exalted to heaven, will be brought down to Hades; for if the mighty works which were done in you had been done in Sodom, it would have remained until this day. But I say to you that it shall be more tolerable for the land of Sodom in the day of judgment than for you." (Matthew 11:20-24 NKJV)*

"Jesus said to them, "Most assuredly, I say to you, before Abraham was, I AM." (John 8:58 NKJV)*

"These things I have spoken to you, that in Me you may have peace. In the world you will have tribulation; but be of good cheer, I have overcome the world." (John 16:33 NKJV)*

•

Messiah, Jesse's offspring shall Reign:

Old Testament
"There shall come forth a Rod from the stem of Jesse, And a Branch shall grow out of his roots. The Spirit of the LORD shall rest upon Him, The Spirit of wisdom and understanding, The Spirit of counsel and might, The Spirit of knowledge and of the fear of the LORD." (Isaiah 11:1,2 NKJV)*

New Testament
"Now Jesus Himself began His ministry at about thirty years of age, being (as was supposed) the son of Joseph, the son (in law) of Heli, the son of Matthat,the son of Levi, the son of Melchi, the son of Janna, the son of Joseph, the son of Mattathiah, the son of Amos, the son of Nahum, the son of Esli, the son of Naggai, the son of Maath, the son of Mattathiah, the son of Semei, the son of Joseph, the son of Judah, the son of Joannas, the son of Rhesa, the son of Zerubbabel, the son of Shealtiel, the son of Neri, the son of Melchi, the son of Addi, the son of Cosam, the son of Elmodam, the son of Er, the son of Jose, the son of Eliezer, the son of Jorim, the son of Matthat, the son of Levi, the son of Simeon, the son of Judah, the son of Joseph, the son of Jonan, the son of Eliakim, the son of Melea, the son of Menan, the son of Mattathah, the son of Nathan, the son of David, the son of Jesse,"(Luke 3:22-32 NKJV) (Lineage of Mary)

•

The Gentiles shall seek Him:

Old Testament
"And in that day there shall be a Root of Jesse, Who shall stand as a banner to the people; For the Gentiles shall seek Him, And His resting place shall be glorious." (Isaiah 11:10 NKJV)*

"For this reason the people also met Him, because they heard that He had done this sign. The Pharisees therefore said among themselves, "You see that you are accomplishing nothing. Look, the world has gone after Him!" (John 12:18,19 NKJV)*

•

Reign in truth and mercy:

Old Testament
"In mercy the throne will be established; And One will sit on it in truth, in the tabernacle of David, Judging and seeking justice and hastening righteousness." (Isaiah 16:4 NKJV)*

New Testament
"He will be great, and will be called the Son of the Highest; and the Lord God will give Him the throne of His father David. And He will reign over the house of Jacob forever, and of His kingdom there will be no end." (Luke 1:32,33 NKJV)*

•

Messiah shall be holder of the keys to the house of David:

Old Testament
"....I will commit your responsibility into his hand. He shall be a father to the inhabitants of Jerusalem And to the house of Judah. The key of the house of David I will lay on his shoulder; So he shall open, and no one shall shut; And he shall shut, and no one shall open." (Isaiah 22:21,22 NKJV)*

New Testament
"And to the angel of the church in Philadelphia write, 'These things says He who is holy, He who is true, "He who has the key of David, He who opens and no one shuts, and shuts and no one opens":" (Revelation 3:7 NKJV)*

•

Messiah will destroy dealth:

Old Testament
"He will swallow up death forever, And the Lord GOD will wipe away tears from all faces; The rebuke of His people He will take away from all the earth; For the LORD has spoken." (Isaiah 25:8 NKJV)*

New Testament
"So when this corruptible has put on incorruption, and this mortal has put on immortality, then shall be brought to pass the saying that is written: "Death is swallowed up in victory." "O Death, where is your sting? O Hades, where is your victory?" (1 Corinthians 15:54 NKJV)*

•

Power over the resurrection of the dead:

Old Testament
"Your dead shall live; Together with my dead body they shall arise. Awake and sing, you who dwell in dust; For your dew is like the dew of herbs, And the earth shall cast out the dead." (Isaiah 26:19 NKJV)*

New Testament
"....Lord, by this time there is a stench, for he has been dead four days." Jesus said to her, "Did I not say to you that if you would believe you would see the glory of God?" Then they took away the stone from the place where the dead man was lying. And Jesus lifted up His eyes and said, "Father, I thank You that You have heard Me. And I know that You always hear Me, but because of the people who are standing by I said this, that they may believe that You sent Me." Now when He had said these things, He cried with a loud voice, "Lazarus, come forth!" And he who had died came out bound hand and foot with graveclothes, and his face was wrapped with a cloth. Jesus said to them, "Loose him, and let him go." (John 11:39-44 NKJV)*

•

Commandments of men put over God's commandments:

Old Testament
"Therefore the Lord said: "Inasmuch as these people draw near with their mouths And honor Me with their lips, But have removed their hearts far from Me, And their fear toward Me is taught by the commandment of men," (Isaiah 29:13 NKJV)*

New Testament
Thus you have made the commandment of God of no effect by your tradition. Hypocrites! Well did Isaiah prophesy about you, saying: 'These people draw near to Me with their mouth, And honor Me with their lips, But their heart is far from Me. And in vain they worship Me, Teaching as doctrines the commandments of men.'" (Matthew 15:7-9 NKJV)*

•

Wisdom of the wise to perish:

Old Testament
"Therefore, behold, I will again do a marvelous work Among this people, A marvelous work and a wonder; For the wisdom of their wise men shall perish, And the understanding of their prudent men shall be hidden." (Isaiah 29:14 NKJV)*

New Testament
"For the message of the cross is foolishness to those who are perishing, but to us who are being saved it is the power of God. For it is written: "I will destroy the wisdom of the wise, And bring to nothing the understanding of the prudent." Where is the wise? Where is the scribe? Where is the disputer of this age? Has not God made foolish the wisdom of this world? For since, in the wisdom of God, the world through wisdom did not know God, it pleased God through the foolishness of the message preached to save those who believe. For Jews request a sign, and Greeks seek after wisdom; but we preach Christ crucified, to the Jews a stumbling block and to the Greeks foolishness, but to those who are called, both Jews and Greeks, Christ the power of God and the wisdom of God. Because the foolishness of God is wiser than men, and the weakness of God is stronger than men." (1 Corinthians 1:18-25 NKJV)*

•

Messiah shall have a Ministry of Miracles:

Old Testament
"Say to those who are fearful-hearted, "Be strong, do not fear! Behold, your God will come with vengeance, With the recompense of God; He will come and save you." Then the eyes of the blind shall be opened, And the ears of the deaf shall be unstopped. Then the lame shall leap like a deer, And the tongue of the dumb sing. For waters shall burst forth in the wilderness, And streams in the desert." (Isaiah 35:4-6 NKJV)*

New Testament
"When He had said these things, He spat on the ground and made clay with the saliva; and He anointed the eyes of the blind man with the clay. And He said to him, "Go, wash in the pool of Siloam" (which is translated, Sent). So he went and washed, and came back seeing." (John 9:6,7 NKJV)*

"Then they brought to Him one who was deaf and had an impediment in his speech, and they begged Him to put His hand on him. And He took him aside from the multitude, and put His fingers in his ears, and He spat and touched his tongue. Then, looking up to heaven, He sighed, and said to him, "Ephphatha," that is, "Be opened." Immediately his ears were opened, and the impediment of his tongue was loosed, and he spoke plainly." (Mark 7:32-36 NKJV)*

"Now a certain man was there who had an infirmity thirty-eight years. When Jesus saw him lying there, and knew that he already had been in that condition a long time, He said to him, "Do you want to be made well?" The sick man answered Him, "Sir, I have no man to put me into the pool when the water is stirred up; but while I am coming, another steps down before me." Jesus said to him, "Rise, take up your bed and walk." And immediately the man was made well, took up his bed, and walked." (John 5:5-7 NKJV)*

•

Messiah to be preceded by one crying in the wilderness: (John the Baptist)

Old Testament

"The voice of one crying in the wilderness: "Prepare the way of the LORD; Make straight in the desert A highway for our God." (Isaiah 40:3,4 NKJV)*

New Testament

"Now this is the testimony of John, when the Jews sent priests and Levites from Jerusalem to ask him, "Who are you?" He confessed, and did not deny, but confessed, "I am not the Christ." And they asked him, "What then? Are you Elijah?" He said, "I am not." "Are you the Prophet?" And he answered, "No." Then they said to him, "Who are you, that we may give an answer to those who sent us? What do you say about yourself?" He said: "I am ' The voice of one crying in the wilderness:" Make straight the way of the LORD,"' as the prophet Isaiah said." (John1:19-23 NKJV)*

•

Crier's pronouncement of Messiah:

Old Testament

"O Zion, You who bring good tidings, Get up into the high mountain; O Jerusalem, You who bring good tidings, Lift up your voice with strength, Lift it up, be not afraid; Say to the cities of Judah, "Behold your God!" (Isaiah 40:9 NKJV)*

New Testament

"Again, the next day, John stood with two of his disciples. And looking at Jesus as He walked, he said, "Behold the Lamb of God!" (John 1:35-36 NKJV)*

•

Messiah to be a Shepherd:

"He will feed His flock like a shepherd; He will gather the lambs with His arm, And carry them in His bosom, And gently lead those who are with young." (Isaiah 40:11 NKJV)*

"The thief does not come except to steal, and to kill, and to destroy. I have come that they may have life, and that they may have it more abundantly. "I am the good shepherd. The good shepherd gives His life for the sheep. But a hireling, he who is not the shepherd, one who does not own the sheep, sees the wolf coming and leaves the sheep and flees; and the wolf catches the sheep and scatters them. The hireling flees because he is a hireling and does not care about the sheep. I am the good shepherd; and I know My sheep, and am known by My own. As the Father knows Me, even so I know the Father; and I lay down My life for the sheep. And other sheep I have which are not of this fold; them also I must bring, and they will hear My voice; and there will be one flock and one shepherd. "Therefore My Father loves Me, because I lay down My life that I may take it again. No one takes it from Me, but I lay it down of Myself. I have power to lay it down, and I have power to take it again." (John 10:10-18 NKJV)*

•

Messiah is God's servant:

"Behold! My Servant whom I uphold, My Elect One in whom My soul delights! I have put My Spirit upon Him; He will bring forth justice to the Gentiles. He will not cry out, nor raise His voice, Nor cause His voice to be heard in the street. A bruised reed He will not break, And smoking flax He will not quench; He will bring forth justice for truth. He will not fail nor be discouraged, Till He has established justice in the earth; And the coastlands shall wait for His law." (Isaiah 40:1-4 NKJV)*

"Behold! My Servant whom I have chosen,My Beloved in whom My soul is well pleased! I will put My Spirit upon Him, And He will declare justice

to the Gentiles.He will not quarrel nor cry out, Nor will anyone hear His voice in the streets. A bruised reed He will not break, And smoking flax He will not quench, Till He sends forth justice to victory; And in His name Gentiles will trust." (Matthew 12:18-21 NKJV)*

•

No other Savior:

Old Testament
"I, even I, am the LORD, And besides Me there is no savior." (Isaiah 43:11 NKJV)*

New Testament
"Nor is there salvation in any other, for there is no other name under heaven given among men by which we must be saved." (Acts 4:12 NKJV)*

•

The Spirit will be poured out:

Old Testament
"For I will pour water on him who is thirsty, And floods on the dry ground; I will pour My Spirit on your descendants, And My blessing on your offspring (Isaiah 44:3NKJV)*

New Testament
"Nevertheless I tell you the truth. It is to your advantage that I go away; for if I do not go away, the Helper will not come to you; but if I depart, I will send Him to you. And when He has come, He will convict the world of sin, and of righteousness, and of judgment: of sin, because they do not believe in Me; of righteousness, because go to My Father and you see Me no more; of judgment, because the ruler of this world is judged. "I still have many things to say to you, but you cannot bear them now. However, when He, the Spirit of truth, has come, He will guide you into all truth; for He will not speak on His own authority, but whatever He hears He will speak; and He will tell you things to come. He will glorify Me, for He will take of what is Mine and declare it to you. All things that

the Father has are Mine. Therefore I said that He will take of Mine and declare it to you.' (John 16:7-15 NKJV)*

•

Messiah shall Judge:

Old Testament

"I have sworn by Myself; The word has gone out of My mouth in righteousness, And shall not return, That to Me every knee shall bow, Every tongue shall take an oath." (Isaiah 45:23 NKJV)*

"He will bring justice to the poor of the people; He will save the children of the needy, And will break in pieces the oppressor"." (Psalm 72:4 NKJV)*

New Testament

"For the Father judges no one, but has committed all judgment to the Son." (John 5:22 NKJV)*

"For it is written: "As I live, says the LORD Every knee shall bow to Me, And every tongue shall confess to God." (Romans. 14:11 NKJV)*

"because He has appointed a day on which He will judge the world in righteousness by the Man whom He has ordained. He has given assurance of this to all by raising Him from the dead." (Acts 17:31 NKJV)*

•

Messiah shall be the first and the last:

Old Testament

" Listen to Me, O Jacob, And Israel, My called: I am He, I am the First, I am also the Last." (Isaiah 48:12 NKJV)*

I have been established from everlasting, From the beginning, before there was ever an earth." (Proverbs 8:23 NKJV)*

New Testament
"This is He of whom I said, 'After me comes a Man who is preferred before me, for He was before me.'" (John 1:30 NKJV)*

"I am the Alpha and the Omega, the Beginning and the End," says the Lord,"who is and who was and who is to come, the Almighty." (Revelation 1:8 NKJV)*

"And when I saw Him, I fell at His feet as dead. But He laid His right hand on me, saying to me, "Do not be afraid; I am the First and the Last." (Revelation 1:17 NKJV)*

"And to the angel of the church of the Laodiceans write, 'These things says the Amen, the Faithful and True Witness, the Beginning of the creation of God:" (Revelation 3:14 NKJV)*

•

Messiah shall be a Teacher:

Old Testament
Thus says the LORD, your Redeemer, The Holy One of Israel: " I am the LORD you God, Who teaches you to profit, Who leads you by the way you should go." (Isaiah 48:17 NKJV)*

New Testament
This man came to Jesus by night and said to Him, "Rabbi, we know that You are a teacher come from God; for no one can do these signs that You do unless God is with him." (John 3:2 NKJV)*

•

Messiah comes from the womb of woman to serve:

Old Testament
"Listen, O coastlands, to Me, And take heed, you peoples from afar! The LORD has called Me from the womb; From the matrix of My mother He has made mention of My name." (Isaiah 49:1 NKJV)*

" And now the LORD says, Who formed Me from the womb to be His Servant, To bring Jacob back to Him, So that Israel is gathered to

Him (For I shall be glorious in the eyes of the LORD, And My God shall be My strength)," (Isaiah 49:5 NKJV)*

New Testament
Now the birth of Jesus Christ was as follows: After His mother Mary was betrothed to Joseph, before they came together, she was found with child of the Holy Spirit." (Matthew 1:18 NKJV)*

And behold, you will conceive in your womb and bring forth a Son, and shall call His name JESUS." (Lluke 1:31 NKJV)*

"but made Himself of no reputation, taking the form of a bondservant, and coming in the likeness of men." (Philipians 2:7 NKJV)*

•

Israel's and the Gentile's Salvation to the ends of the earth:

Old Testament
"Indeed He says, ' It is too small a thing that You should be My Servant To raise up the tribes of Jacob, And to restore the preserved ones of Israel; I will also give You as a light to the Gentiles, That You should be My salvation to the ends of the earth.'" (Isaih 49:6 NKJV)*

New Testament
"Lord, now You are letting Your servant depart in peace, According to Your word; For my eyes have seen Your salvation Which You have prepared before the face of all peoples, A light to bring revelation to the Gentiles, And the glory of Your people Israel." (Luke 2:29-32 NKJV)*

"For so the Lord has commanded us: ' I have set you as a light to the Gentiles That you should be for salvation to the ends of the earth.'" (Acts 13:47 NKJV)*

"And when there had been much dispute, Peter rose up and said to them: "Men and brethren, you know that a good while ago God chose among us, that by my mouth the Gentiles should hear the word of the gospel and believe. So God, who knows the heart, acknowledged them by giving them the Holy Spirit, just as He did to us,"
(Acts 15:7,8 NKJV)*

•

Messiah despised of man, hated by the Nation:

Old Testament
"Thus says the LORD, The Redeemer of Israel, their Holy One, To Him whom man despises, To Him whom the nation abhors, To the Servant of rulers:" (Isaiah 49:7 NKJV)*

New Testament
"Then the Jews answered and said to Him, "Do we not say rightly that You are a Samaritan and have a demon?" Jesus answered, "I do not have a demon; but I honor My Father, and you dishonor Me." (John 8:48-49 NKJV)*

•

Blackness (an eclipse) sets in at Messiah's humiliation:

Old Testament
"I clothe the heavens with blackness, And I make sackcloth their covering." (Isaiah 50:3 NKJV)*

New Testament
"Now it was about the sixth hour, and there was darkness over all the earth until the ninth hour. Then the sun was darkened, and the veil of the temple was torn in two." (Luke 23:44,45 NKJV)*

•

Messiah a counselor of God:

Old Testament
"The Lord GOD has given Me The tongue of the learned, That I should know how to speak A word in season to him who is weary. He awakens Me morning by morning, He awakens My ear To hear as the learned." (Isaiah 50:4 NKJV)*

"Come to Me, all you who labor and are heavy laden, and I will give you rest. Take My yoke upon you and learn from Me, for I am gentle and lowly in heart, and you will find rest for your souls." (Matthew 11:28,29 NKJV)*

•

Messiah was bound willingly to serve:

Old Testament
"The Lord GOD has opened My ear; And I was not rebellious, Nor did I turn away." (Isaiah 50:5 NKJV)*

New Testament
He went a little farther and fell on His face, and prayed, saying, "O My Father, if it is possible, let this cup pass from Me; nevertheless, not as I will, but as You will." (Matthew 26:39 NKJV)*

•

Messiah gave His back to the smiters; His beard plucked:

Old Testament
I gave My back to those who struck Me, And My cheeks to those who plucked out the beard; I did not hide My face from shame and spitting." (Isaiah 50:6 NKJV)*

New Testament
Then he released Barabbas to them; and when he had scourged Jesus, he delivered Him to be crucified." (Matthew 27:26 NKJV)*

"Then they spat on Him, and took the reed and struck Him on the head. (Matthew 27:30 NKJV)*

"Then they spat in His face and beat Him; and others struck Him with the palms of their hands, (Matthew 26:67 NKJV)*

•

Messiah proclaims peace, glad tidings and salvation and lifts God up:

Old Testament

"How beautiful upon the mountains Are the feet of him who brings good news, Who proclaims peace, Who brings glad tidings of good things, Who proclaims salvation, Who says to Zion, " Your God reigns!" (Isaiah 52:7 NKJV)*

New Testament

Then Jesus returned in the power of the Spirit to Galilee, and news of Him went out through the entire surrounding region. And He taught in their synagogues, being glorified by all." (Luke 4:14-15 NKJV)*

".....Now it came to pass, afterward, that He went through every city and village, preaching and bringing the glad tidings of the kingdom of God. And the twelve were with Him." (Luke 8:1 NKJV)*

•

Messiah, God's exalted servant shall deal prudently:

Old Testament

Behold, My Servant shall deal prudently; He shall be exalted and extolled and be very high." (Isaiah 52:13 NKJV)*

New Testament

Now when He had spoken these things, while they watched, He was taken up, and a cloud received Him out of their sight. And while they looked steadfastly toward heaven as He went up, behold, two men stood by them in white apparel, who also said, "Men of Galilee, why do you stand gazing up into heaven? This same Jesus, who was taken up from you into heaven, will so come in like manner as you saw Him go into heaven." (Acts 1:9-11 NKJV)*

"..and what is the exceeding greatness of His power toward us who believe, according to the working of His mighty power which He worked in Christ when He raised Him from the dead and seated Him at His right hand in the heavenly places, far above all principality and power and might and dominion, and every name that is named, not only in this age

but also in that which is to come. And He put all things under His feet, and gave Him to be head over all things to the church." (Ephesians 1:19-22 NKJV)*

"Let this mind be in you which was also in Christ Jesus, who, being in the form of God, did not consider it robbery to be equal with God, but made Himself of no reputation, taking the form of a bondservant, and coming in the likeness of men. And being found in appearance as a man, He humbled Himself and became obedient to the point of death, even the death of the cross. Therefore God also has highly exalted Him and given Him the name which is above every name, that at the name of Jesus every knee should bow, of those in heaven, and of those on earth, and of those under the earth, and that every tongue should confess that Jesus Christ is Lord, to the glory of God the Father" (Philipians 2:5-8 NKJV)*

•

Messiah marred more than any man:

Old Testament
"Just as many were astonished at you, So His visage was marred more than any man, And His form more than the sons of men;" (Isaiah 52:14 NKJV)*

New Testament
"Then He took the twelve aside and said to them, "Behold, we are going up to Jerusalem, and all things that are written by the prophets concerning the Son of Man will be accomplished. For He will be delivered to the Gentiles and will be mocked and insulted and spit upon. They will scourge Him and kill Him. And the third day He will rise again." But they understood none of these things; this saying was hidden from them, and they did not know the things which were spoken." (Matthew 26:31-34 NKJV)*

"So Pilate, wanting to gratify the crowd, released Barabbas to them; and he delivered Jesus, after he had scourged Him, to be crucified. Then the soldiers led Him away into the hall called Praetorium, and they called together the whole garrison. And they clothed Him with purple; and they twisted a crown of thorns, put it on His head, and began to salute Him, "Hail, King of the Jews!" Then they struck Him on the head with a reed and spat on Him; and bowing the knee, they worshiped Him. And

when they had mocked Him, they took the purple off Him, put His own clothes on Him, and led Him out to crucify Him." (Mark 15:16-20 NKJV)*

•

Messiah's own people will not believe Him:

Old Testament
"Who has believed our report? And to whom has the arm of the LORD been revealed? (Isaiah 53:1 NKJV)*

New Testament
"But although He had done so many signs before them, they did not believe in Him, that the word of Isaiah the prophet might be fulfilled, which he spoke: "Lord, who has believed our report? And to whom has the arm of the LORD been revealed?"[a] (John 12:37,38 NKJV)*

•

Messiah shall grow up during hard times as an ordinary man:

Old Testament
For He shall grow up before Him as a tender plant, And as a root out of dry ground. He has no form or comeliness; And when we see Him, There is no beauty that we should desire Him." (Isaiah 53:2 NKJV)*

New Testament
"So it was, that while they were there, the days were completed for her to be delivered. And she brought forth her firstborn Son, and wrapped Him in swaddling cloths, and laid Him in a manger, because there was no room for them in the inn." (Luke 2:6-7 NKJV)*

"but made Himself of no reputation, taking the form of a bondservant, and coming in the likeness of men. And being found in appearance as a man, He humbled Himself and became obedient to the point of death, even the death of the cross." (Philipians 2:7-8 NKJV)*

•

Men conceal their association with Messiah; they reject and despise Him, a man of sorrow:

Old Testament
"He is despised and rejected by men, A Man of sorrows and acquainted with grief. And we hid, as it were, our faces from Him; He was despised, and we did not esteem Him." (Isaiah 53:3 NKJV)*

New Testament
"So all those in the synagogue, when they heard these things, were filled with wrath, and rose up and thrust Him out of the city; and they led Him to the brow of the hill on which their city was built, that they might throw Him down over the cliff. Then passing through the midst of them, He went His way." (Luke 4:28-30 NKJV)*

"........Then all the disciples forsook Him and fled." (Matthew 26:56 NKJV)*

"Now Simon Peter stood and warmed himself. Therefore they said to him, "You are not also one of His disciples, are you?" He denied it and said, "I am not!" One of the servants of the high priest, a relative of him whose ear Peter cut off, said, "Did I not see you in the garden with Him?" Peter then denied again; and immediately a rooster crowed." (John 18:25-27 NKJV)*

"The governor answered and said to them, "Which of the two do you want me to release to you?" They said, "Barabbas!" Pilate said to them, "What then shall I do with Jesus who is called Christ?" They all said to him, "Let Him be crucified!" Then the governor said, "Why, what evil has He done?" But they cried out all the more, saying, "Let Him be crucified!" (Matthew 27:21-23 NKJV)*

"Now as He drew near, He saw the city and wept over it, saying, "If you had known, even you, especially in this your day, the things that make for your peace! But now they are hidden from your eyes." (Luke 19:41-42 NKJV)*

•

Messiah is assessed as stricken of God, He bore our sins and sorrows:

Old Testament
"Surely He has borne our griefs And carried our sorrows; Yet we esteemed Him stricken, Smitten by God, and afflicted." (Isaiah 53:4 NKJV)*

New Testament
"who Himself bore our sins in His own body on the tree, that we, having died to sins, might live for righteousness—by whose stripes you were healed." (1 Peter 2:24 NKJV)*

"And He came down with them and stood on a level place with a crowd of His disciples and a great multitude of people from all Judea and Jerusalem, and from the seacoast of Tyre and Sidon, who came to hear Him and be healed their diseases, as well as those who were tormented with unclean spirits. And they were healed. And the whole multitude sought to touch Him, for power went out from Him and healed them all." (Luke 6:17-19 NKJV)*

Likewise the chief priests also, mocking with the scribes and elders, said, "He saved others; Himself He cannot save. If He is the King of Israel, let Him now come down from the cross, and we will believe Him." (Luke 27:41-42 NKJV)*

•

Messiah takes upon Himself the penalty for mankind for our peace with God:

Old Testament
But He was wounded for our transgressions, He was bruised for our iniquities; The chastisement for our peace was upon Him, And by His stripes we are healed." (Isaiah 53:5 NKJV)*

New Testament
And when they had come to the place called Calvary, there they crucified Him, and the criminals, one on the right hand and the other on the left." (Luke 23:33 NKJV)*

•

God laid the sin for all mankind on Messiah.

Old Testament

All we like sheep have gone astray; We have turned, every one, to his own way; And the LORD has laid on Him the iniquity of us all" (Isaiah 53:6 NKJV)*

New Testament

"who gave Himself for our sins, that He might deliver us from this present evil age, according to the will of our God and Father," (Galatians 1:4 NKJV)*

In this is love, not that we loved God, but that He loved us and sent His Son to be the propitiation for our sins." (1 John 4:10 NKJV)*

•

He would be oppressed and afflicted yet kept silent as a sheep to the slaughter:

Old Testament

He was oppressed and He was afflicted, Yet He opened not His mouth; He was led as a lamb to the slaughter, And as a sheep before its shearers is silent, So He opened not His mouth." (Isaiah 53:7 NKJV)*

New Testament

"And while He was being accused by the chief priests and elders, He answered nothing. Then Pilate said to Him, "Do You not hear how many things they testify against You?" But He answered him not one word, so that the governor marveled greatly." (Matthew 27:12-14 NKJV)*

Then the soldiers of the governor took Jesus into the Praetorium and gathered the whole garrison around Him. And they stripped Him and put a scarlet robe on Him. When they had twisted a crown of thorns, they put it on His head, and a reed in His right hand. And they bowed the knee before Him and mocked Him, saying, "Hail, King of the Jews!" Then they spat on Him, and took the reed and struck Him on the head. And when they had mocked Him, they took the robe off Him, put His own

271

clothes on Him, and led Him away to be crucified." (Matthew 27: 27-31 NKJV)*

•

Messiah was imprisoned, judged, and killed for our sins:

Old Testament
He was taken from prison and from judgment, And who will declare His generation? For He was cut off from the land of the living; For the transgressions of *My people He was stricken." (Isaiah 53:8 NKJV)**

New Testament
"And those who had laid hold of Jesus led Him away to Caiaphas the high priest, where the scribes and the elders were assembled." (Matthew 26:57 NKJV)*

"And when they had mocked Him, they took the robe off Him, put His own clothes on Him, and led Him away to be crucified." (Matthew 27:31 NKJV)*

"Pilate then went out to them and said, "What accusation do you bring against this Man?" They answered and said to him, "If He were not an evildoer, we would not have delivered Him up to you." Then Pilate said to them, "You take Him and judge Him according to your law." Therefore the Jews said to him, "It is not lawful for us to put anyone to death," (John 18:29-31 NKJV)*

"Then they crucified Him, and divided His garments, casting lots, that it might be fulfilled which was spoken by the prophet: "They divided My garments among them, And for My clothing they cast lots." (Matthew 27:35 NKJV)*

And He Himself is the propitiation for our sins, and not for ours only but also for the whole world." (1 John2:2 NKJV)*

•

Messiah is permitted to be buried in a rich man's grave because He had not done violence and had spoken no deceit:

Old Testament
"And they made His grave with the wicked—But with the rich at His death, Because He had done no violence, Nor *was any* deceit in His mouth." (Isaiah 53:9 NKJV)*

New Testament
"Now when evening had come, there came a rich man from Arimathea, named Joseph, who himself had also become a disciple of Jesus. This man went to Pilate and asked for the body of Jesus. Then Pilate commanded the body to be given to him. When Joseph had taken the body, he wrapped it in a clean linen cloth, and laid it in his new tomb which he had hewn out of the rock; and he rolled a large stone against the door of the tomb, and departed."(Matthew 27:57-61 NKJV)*

"And the chief priests accused Him of many things, but He answered nothing." (Mark 15:3 NKJV)*

"Pilate said to Him, "What is truth?" And when he had said this, he went out again to the Jews, and said to them, "I find no fault in Him at all." (John 18:38 NKJV)*

•

God's will that Messiah die for mankind as an offering for sin:

Old Testament
"Yet it pleased the LORD to bruise Him; He has put Him to grief. When You make His soul an offering for sin, He shall see His seed, He shall prolong His days, And the pleasure of the LORD shall prosper in His hand." (Isaiah 53:10 NKJV)*

New Testament
"So Jesus said to Peter, "Put your sword into the sheath. Shall I not drink the cup which My Father has given Me?" (John 18:11 NKJV)*

"...just as the Son of Man did not come to be served, but to serve, and to give His life a ransom for many." (Matthew 20:28 NKJV)*

"He who believes and is baptized will be saved; but he who does not believe will be condemned." (Mark 16:16 NKJV)*

"Jesus spoke these words, lifted up His eyes to heaven, and said: "Father, the hour has come. Glorify Your Son, that Your Son also may glorify You, as You have given Him authority over all flesh, that He should give eternal life to as many as You have given Him. And this is eternal life, that they may know You, the only true God, and Jesus Christ whom You have sent. I have glorified You on the earth. I have finished the work which You have given Me to do. And now, O Father, glorify Me together with Yourself, with the glory which I had with You before the world was." (John17:1-5 NKJV)*

•

Messiah's suffering and death shall provide full satisfaction to God for our sin:

Old Testament
"He shall see the labor of His soul, and be satisfied. By His knowledge My righteous Servant shall justify many, For He shall bear their iniquities." (Isaiah 53:11 NKJV)*

New Testament
"Now My soul is troubled, and what shall I say? 'Father, save Me from this hour'? But for this purpose I came to this hour." (John 12:27 NKJV)*

"But God demonstrates His own love toward us, in that while we were still sinners, Christ died for us. Much more then, having now been justified by His blood, we shall be saved from wrath through Him." (Romans 5:8-9 NKJV)*

"Therefore, as through one man's offense judgment came to all men, resulting in condemnation, even so through one Man's righteous act the free gift came to all men, resulting in justification of life. For as by one man's disobedience many were made sinners, so also by one Man's obedience many will be made righteous." (Romans 5:18-19 NKJV)*

"And He Himself is the propitiation for our sins, and not for ours only but also for the whole world." (1 John 2:2 NKJV)*

"so Christ was offered once to bear the sins of many. To those who eagerly wait for Him He will appear a second time, apart from sin, for salvation." (Hebrews 9:28 NKJV)*

•

Exalted for His sacrifice, Messiah would be grouped with criminals and give up His life to save mankind making intercession for the transgressors:

Old Testament

Therefore I will divide Him a portion with the great, And He shall divide the spoil with the strong, Because He poured out His soul unto death, And He was numbered with the transgressors, And He bore the sin of many, And made intercession for the transgressors." (Isaiah 53:12 NKJV)*

New Testament

And Jesus came and spoke to them, saying, "All authority has been given to Me in heaven and on earth." (Matthew 28:18 NKJV)*

There were also two others, criminals, led with Him to be put to death." (Luke 23:32 NKJV)*

Then Jesus said, "Father, forgive them, for they do not know what they do."And they divided His garments and cast lots." (Luke 23:34 NKJV)*

And when Jesus had cried out with a loud voice, He said, "Father, 'into Your hands I commit My spirit.'"Having said this, He breathed His last." (Luke 23:46 NKJV)*

For He made Him who knew no sin to be sin for us, that we might become the righteousness of God in Him." (2 Corinthians 5:21 NKJV)*

•

Come to Messiah all who thirst:

Old Testament

"Ho! Everyone who thirsts, Come to the waters And you who have no money, Come, buy and eat. Yes, come, buy wine and milk Without money and without price." (Isaiah 55:1 NKJV)*

New Testament
Jesus answered and said to her, "Whoever drinks of this water will thirst again, but whoever drinks of the water that I shall give him will never thirst. But the water that I shall give him will become in him a fountain of water springing up into everlasting life." (John 4:13-14 NKJV)*

•

Messiah the sure mercies of David:

Old Testament
Incline your ear, and come to Me. Hear, and your soul shall live; And I will make an everlasting covenant with you— The sure mercies of David." (Isaiah 55:3 NKJV)*

New Testament
And that He raised Him from the dead, no more to return to corruption, He has spoken thus: ' I will give you the sure mercies of David." (Acts 13:34 NKJV)*

•

Messiah a witness and a leader:

Old Testament
Indeed I have given him as a witness to the people, A leader and commander for the people." (Isaiah 55:4 NKJV)*

New Testament
Pilate therefore said to Him, "Are You a king then?" Jesus answered, "You say rightly that I am a king. For this cause I was born, and for this cause I have come into the world, that I should bear witness to the truth. Everyone who is of the truth hears My voice." (John 18:37 NKJV)*

•

Foreign nations shall come to God because of Messiah:

Old Testament
"Surely you shall call a nation you do not know, And nations who do not know you shall run to you, Because of the LORD your God, And the Holy One of Israel; For He has glorified you." (Isaiah 55:5 NKJV)*

New Testament
"And this gospel of the kingdom will be preached in all the world as a witness to all the nations, and then the end will come." (Matthew 24:14 NKJV)*

"Through Him we have received grace and apostleship for obedience to the faith among all nations for His name" (Romans 1:5 NKJV)*

"Now when they had come and gathered the church together, they reported all that God had done with them, and that He had opened the door of faith to the Gentiles." (Acts 14:27 NKJV)*

•

God's arm would come equipped with righteousness and zeal to provide salvation:

Old Testament
"He saw that there was no man, And wondered that there was no intercessor; Therefore His own arm brought salvation for Him; And His own righteousness, it sustained Him. For He put on righteousness as a breastplate, And a helmet of salvation on His head; He put on the garments of vengeance for clothing, And was clad with zeal as a cloak." (Isaiah 59:15-17 NKJV)*

New Testament
"And this is the will of Him who sent Me, that everyone who sees the Son and believes in Him may have everlasting life; and I will raise him up at the last day." (John 6:40 NKJV)*

"Therefore whoever confesses Me before men, him I will also confess before My Father who is in heaven." (Matthew 10:32 NKJV)*

'For there is one God and one Mediator between God and men, the Man Christ Jesus " (1 Timothy 2:5 NKJV)*

•

Messiah would come to Zion as Redeemer:

Old Testament
"The Redeemer will come to Zion, And to those who turn from transgression in Jacob," Says the LORD." (Isaiah 59:20 NKJV)*

New Testament
"And coming in that instant she gave thanks to the Lord, and spoke of Him to all those who looked for redemption in Jerusalem." (Luke2:38 NKJV)*

•

Nations shall walk in the light because of Messiah:

Old Testament
"Arise, shine; For your light has come! And the glory of the LORD is risen upon you. For behold, the darkness shall cover the earth, And deep darkness the people; But the LORD will arise over you, And His glory will be seen upon you. The Gentiles shall come to your light, And kings to the brightness of your rising." (Isaiah 60:1-3 NKJV)*

New Testament
"A light to bring revelation to the Gentiles, And the glory of Your people Israel." (Luke 2:32 NKJV)*

•

The Spirit of God is upon Messiah:

Old Testament
"The Spirit of the Lord GOD is upon Me, Because the LORD has anointed Me To preach good tidings to the poor; He has sent Me to heal the brokenhearted, To proclaim liberty to the captives, And the opening of the prison to those who are bound; To proclaim the acceptable year of the LORD, And the day of vengeance of our God; To comfort all who mourn," (Isaiah 61:1-2 NKJV)*

New Testament

"When He had been baptized, Jesus came up immediately from the water; and behold, the heavens were opened to Him, and He saw the Spirit of God descending like a dove and alighting upon Him. And suddenly a voice came from heaven, saying, "This is My beloved Son, in whom I am well pleased." (Matthew 3:16 NKJV)*

•

Messiah would preach the good news of freedom from sin and bondage and proclaim a period of grace and the day of vengence:

Old Testament

"The Spirit of the Lord GOD is upon Me, Because the LORD has anointed Me To preach good tidings to the poor; He has sent Me to heal the brokenhearted, To proclaim liberty to the captives, And the opening of the prison to those who are bound; To proclaim the acceptable year of the LORD, And the day of vengeance of our God; To comfort all who mourn," (Isaiah 61:1-2 NKJV)*

New Testament

So He came to Nazareth, where He had been brought up. And as His custom was, He went into the synagogue on the Sabbath day, and stood up to read. ¹⁷ And He was handed the book of the prophet Isaiah. And when He had opened the book, He found the place where it was written: " The Spirit of the LORD is upon Me, Because He has anointed Me To preach the gospel to the poor; He has sent Me to heal the broken-hearted, To proclaim liberty to the captive And recovery of sight to the blind, To set at liberty those who are oppressed; To proclaim the acceptable year of the LORD." Then He closed the book, and gave it back to the attendant and sat down. And the eyes of all who were in the synagogue were fixed on Him. ²¹ And He began to say to them, "Today this Scripture is fulfilled in your hearing." (Luke 4:16-21 NKJV)*

•

Messiah called by a new name:

Old Testament
"For Zion's sake I will not hold My peace, And for Jerusalem's sake I will not rest, Until her righteousness goes forth as brightness, And her salvation as a lamp that burns. The Gentiles shall see your righteousness, And all kings your glory. You shall be called by a new name, Which the mouth of the LORD will name." (Isaiah 62:1-2 NKJV)*

New Testament
"A light to bring revelation to the Gentiles, And the glory of Your people Israel." (Luke 2:32 NKJV*

"He who overcomes, I will make him a pillar in the temple of My God, and he shall go out no more. I will write on him the name of My God and the name of the city of My God, the New Jerusalem, which comes down out of heaven from My God. And I will write on him My new name." (Revelation 3:12 NKJV)*

•

King Messiah enters Jerusalem on a Colt:

Old Testament
"Rejoice greatly, O daughter of Zion! Shout, O daughter of Jerusalem! Behold, your King is coming to you; He is just and having salvation, Lowly and riding on a donkey, A colt, the foal of a donkey." (Zechariah 9:9 NKJV)*

New Testament
They brought the donkey and the colt, laid their clothes on them, and set Him on them. And a very great multitude spread their clothes on the road; others cut down branches from the trees and spread them on the road. Then the multitudes who went before and those who followed cried out, saying: "Hosanna to the Son of David! ' Blessed is He who comes in the name of the LORD!'Hosanna in the highest!" And when He had come into Jerusalem, all the city was moved, saying "Who is this?" So the multitudes said, "This is Jesus, the prophet from Nazareth of Galilee." (Matthew 21:7-11 NKJV)*

●

Messiah does it alone, His robe with blood:

Old Testament

"Who is this who comes from Edom, With dyed garments from Bozrah, This One who is glorious in His apparel, Traveling in the greatness of His strength? — "I who speak in righteousness, mighty to save." Why is Your apparel red, And Your garments like one who treads in the winepress? "I have trodden the winepress alone, And from the peoples no one was with Me. For I have trodden them in My anger, And trampled them in My fury; Their blood is sprinkled upon My garments, And I have stained all My robes.' (Isaiah 63:1-3 NKJV)*

New Testament

"He was clothed with a robe dipped in blood, and His name is called The Word of God." (Revelation 19:13 NKJV)*

●

Messiah is afflicted with the afflicted:

Old Testament

For He said, "Surely they are My people, Children who will not lie." So He became their Savior. In all their affliction He was afflicted, And the Angel of His Presence saved them; In His love and in His pity He redeemed them; And He bore them and carried them All the days of old." (Isaiah 63:8-9 NKJV)*

New Testament

Then the King will say to those on His right hand, 'Come, you blessed of My Father, inherit the kingdom prepared for you from the foundation of the world: for I was hungry and you gave Me food; I was thirsty and you gave Me drink; I was a stranger and you took Me in; I was naked and you clothed Me; I was sick and you visited Me; I was in prison and you came to Me.' "Then the righteous will answer Him, saying, 'Lord, when did we see You hungry and feed You, or thirsty and give You drink? When did we see You a stranger and take You in, or naked and clothe You? Or when did we see You sick, or in prison, and come to You?' And the King will answer and say to them, 'Assuredly, I say to you, inasmuch as you

did it to one of the least of these My brethren, you did it to Me.'"
(Matthew 25:34-40 NKJV)*

•

God's New Heaven and New Earth, the eternal place for His righteous people:

Old Testament

"For behold, I create new heavens and a new earth; And the former shall not be remembered or come to mind. But be glad and rejoice forever in what I create; For behold, I create Jerusalem as a rejoicing, And her people a joy. I will rejoice in Jerusalem, And joy in My people; The voice of weeping shall no longer be heard in her, Nor the voice of crying." (Isaiah 65:17-25 NKJV)*

New Testament

"Now I saw a new heaven and a new earth, for the first heaven and the first earth had passed away. Also there was no more sea. Then I, John, saw the holy city, New Jerusalem, coming down out of heaven from God, prepared as a bride adorned for her husband. And I heard a loud voice from heaven saying, "Behold, the tabernacle of God is with men, and He will dwell with them, and they shall be His people. God Himself will be with them and be their God. And God will wipe away every tear from their eyes; there shall be no more death, nor sorrow, nor crying. There shall be no more pain, for the former things have passed away." (Revelation21:1-4 NKJV)*

"Nevertheless we, according to His promise, look for new heavens and a new earth in which righteousness dwells." (2 Peter 3:13 NKJV)*

•

Messiah a descendant of David:

Old Testament

" Behold, the days are coming," says the LORD, " That I will raise to David a Branch of righteousness; A King shall reign and prosper, And execute judgment and righteousness in the earth." (Jeremiah 23:5 NKJV)*

"'Behold, the days are coming,' says the LORD, 'that I will perform that good thing which I have promised to the house of Israel and to the house of Judah: ' In those days and at that time I will cause to grow up to David A Branch of righteousness; He shall execute judgment and righteousness in the earth." (Jeremiah 33:14-15 NKJV)*

"Thus says the Lord GOD: "I will take also one of the highest branches of the high cedar and set it out. I will crop off from the topmost of its young twigs a tender one, and will plant it on a high and prominent mountain. On the mountain height of Israel I will plant it; and it will bring forth boughs, and bear fruit, and be a majestic cedar. Under it will dwell birds of every sort; in the shadow of its branches they will dwell. And all the trees of the field shall know that I, the LORD, have brought down the high tree and exalted the low tree, dried up the green tree and made the dry tree flourish; I, the LORD, have spoken and have done it." (Ezekiel 17:22-24 NKJV)*

"I will establish one shepherd over them, and he shall feed them—My servant David. He shall feed them and be their shepherd. And I, the LORD, will be their God, and My servant David a prince among them; I, the LORD, have spoken." (Ezekiel 34:23-24 NKJV)*

New Testament

"The book of the genealogy of Jesus Christ, the Son of David, the Son of Abraham:" (Matthew 1:1 NKJV)*

"Now Jesus Himself began His ministry at about thirty years of age, being (as was supposed) the son of Joseph, the son of Heli, the son of Matthat, the son of Levi, the son of Melchi, the son of Janna, the son of Joseph, the son of Mattathiah, the son of Amos, the son of Nahum, the son of Esli, the son of Naggai, the son of Maath, the son of Mattathiah, the son of Semei, the son of Joseph, the son of Judah, the son of Joannas, the son of Rhesa, the son of Zerubbabel, the son of Shealtiel, the son of Neri, the son of Melchi, the son of Addi, the son of Cosam, the son of Elmodam, the son of Er, the son of Jose, the son of Eliezer, the son of Jorim, the son of Matthat, the son of Levi, the son of Simeon, the son of Judah, the son of Joseph, the son of Jonan, the son of Eliakim, the son of Melea, the son of Menan, the son of Mattathah, the son of Nathan, the son of David," (Luke 3:23-31 NKJV)*

•

The Messiah would be God and Man:

Old Testament
"In His days Judah will be saved, And Israel will dwell safely; Now this is His name by which He will be called: THE LORD (YAHVEH) OUR RIGHTEOUSNESS." (Jeremiah 23:6 NKJV)*

New Testament
"You call Me Teacher and Lord, and you say well, for so I am. (John13:13 NKJV)*

"And without controversy great is the mystery of godliness: God was manifested in the flesh, Justified in the Spirit, Seen by angels, Preached among the Gentiles, Believed on in the world, Received up in glory." (1 Timothy 3:16 NKJV)*

•

The Messiah would be born a King:

Old Testament
"But they shall serve the LORD (Yahweh) their God, And David their king, Whom I will raise up for them." (Jeremiah 30:9 NKJV)*

New Testament
"Pilate therefore said to Him, "Are You a king then?" Jesus answered, "You say rightly that I am a king. For this cause I was born, and for this cause I have come into the world, that I should bear witness to the truth. Everyone who is of the truth hears My voice." (John 18:37 NKJV)*

"and from Jesus Christ, the faithful witness, the firstborn from the dead, and the ruler over the kings of the earth. To Him who loved us and washed us from our sins in His own blood," (Revelation 1:5 NKJV)*

•

As in Moses' time, the infants massacred:

Old Testament
"Thus says the LORD: " A voice was heard in Ramah, Lamentation and bitter weeping, Rachel weeping for her children, Refusing to be

comforted for her children, Because they are no more." (Jeremiah 31:15 NKJV)*

New Testament

"Then Herod, when he saw that he was deceived by the wise men, was exceedingly angry; and he sent forth and put to death all the male children who were in Bethlehem and in all its districts, from two years old and under, according to the time which he had determined from the wise men. Then was fulfilled what was spoken by Jeremiah the prophet, saying: " A voice was heard in Rama Lamentation, weeping, and great mourning, Rachel weeping for her children, Refusing to be comforted, Because they are no more." (Matthew 2:16-18 NKJV)*

•

Messiah to be born of a virgin:

Old Testament

"How long will you gad about, O you backsliding daughter? For the LORD has created a new thing in the earth—A woman shall encompass a man." (Jeremiah 31:22 NKJV)*

New Testament

"Now the birth of Jesus Christ was as follows: After His mother Mary was betrothed to Joseph, before they came together, she was found with child of the Holy Spirit. Then Joseph her husband, being a just man, and not wanting to make her a public example, was minded to put her away secretly. But while he thought about these things, behold, an angel of the Lord appeared to him in a dream, saying, "Joseph, son of David, do not be afraid to take to you Mary your wife, for that which is conceived in her is of the Holy Spirit. And she will bring forth a Son, and you shall call His name JESUS, for He will save His people from their sins." So all this was done that it might be fulfilled which was spoken by the Lord through the prophet, saying: "Behold, the virgin shall be with child, and bear a Son, and they shall call His name Immanuel," which is translated, "God with us." (Matthew 1:18-22 NKJV)*

•

The Messiah would be the new covenant:

Old Testament
"Behold, the days are coming, says the LORD, when I will make a new covenant with the house of Israel and with the house of Judah—not according to the covenant that I made with their fathers in the day that I took them by the hand to lead them out of the land of Egypt, My covenant which they broke, though I was a husband to them, says the LORD. But this is the covenant that I will make with the house of Israel after those days, says the LORD: I will put My law in their minds, and write it on their hearts; and I will be their God, and they shall be My people. No more shall every man teach his neighbor, and every man his brother, saying, 'Know the LORD,' for they all shall know Me, from the least of them to the greatest of them, says the LORD. For I will forgive their iniquity, and their sin I will remember no more." (Jeremiah 31:31-34 NKJV)*

New Testament
"For this is My blood of the new covenant, which is shed for many for the remission of sins." (Matthew 26:28 NKJV)*

•

The exalted Messiah has a right to the crown:

Old Testament
"thus says the Lord GOD: " Remove the turban, and take off the crown; Nothing shall remain the same. Exalt the humble, and humble the exalted. Overthrown, overthrown, I will make it overthrown! It shall be no longer, Until He comes whose right it is, And I will give it to Him."' (Ezekiel 21:26-27 NKJV)*

New Testament
"Him God has exalted to His right hand to be Prince and Savior, to give repentance to Israel and forgiveness of sins." (Acts 5:31 NKJV)*

"God, who at various times and in various ways spoke in time past to the fathers by the prophets, [2] has in these last days spoken to us by His Son, whom He has appointed heir of all things, through whom also He made the worlds;" (Luke 1:1-2 NKJV)*

•

Messiah is the stone cut without hands:

Old Testament

"You watched while a stone was cut out without hands, which struck the image on its feet of iron and clay, and broke them in pieces. Then the iron, the clay, the bronze, the silver, and the gold were crushed together, and became like chaff from the summer threshing floors; the wind carried them away so that no trace of them was found. And the stone that struck the image became a great mountain and filled the whole earth." (Daniel 2:34-35 NKJV)*

New Testament

"let it be known to you all, and to all the people of Israel, that by the name of Jesus Christ of Nazareth, whom you crucified, whom God raised from the dead, by Him this man stands here before you whole. This is the 'stone which was rejected by you builders, which has become the chief cornerstone. 'Nor is there salvation in any other, for there is no other name under heaven given among men by which we must be saved." (Acts 4:10-12 NKJV)*

•

The Messiah shall reign over His Triumphant Kingdom:

Old Testament

"And in the days of these kings the God of heaven will set up a kingdom which shall never be destroyed; and the kingdom shall not be left to other people; it shall break in pieces and consume all these kingdoms, and it shall stand forever. Inasmuch as you saw that the stone was cut out of the mountain without hands, and that it broke in pieces the iron, the bronze, the clay, the silver, and the gold—the great God has made known to the king what will come to pass after this. The dream is certain, and its interpretation is sure." (Daniel 2:44-45 NKJV)*

New Testament

"And He will reign over the house of Jacob forever, and of His kingdom there will be no end." (Luke 1:33 NKJV)*

"Then comes the end, when He delivers the kingdom to God the Father, when He puts an end to all rule and all authority and power." (1 Corinthians 15:24 NKJV)*

"Then the seventh angel sounded: And there were loud voices in heaven, saying, "The kingdoms of this world have become the kingdoms of our Lord and of His Christ, and He shall reign forever and ever!" (Revelation 11:15 NKJV)*

•

"The Messiah will come from the clouds of heaven highly exalted whose dominion would be everlasting:

Old Testament

"I was watching in the night visions, And behold, One like the Son of Man, Coming with the clouds of heaven! He came to the Ancient of Days, And they brought Him near before Him. Then to Him was given dominion and glory and a kingdom, That all peoples, nations, and languages should serve Him. His dominion is an everlasting dominion, Which shall not pass away, And His kingdom the one Which shall not be destroyed." (Daniel 7:13-14 NKJV)*

New Testament

"Now when He had spoken these things, while they watched, He was taken up, and a cloud received Him out of their sight. And while they looked steadfastly toward heaven as He went up, behold, two men stood by them in white apparel, who also said, "Men of Galilee, why do you stand gazing up into heaven? This same Jesus, who was taken up from you into heaven, will so come in like manner as you saw Him go into heaven." (Acts 1:9-11 NKJV)*

"and what is the exceeding greatness of His power toward us who believe, according to the working of His mighty power which He worked in Christ when He raised Him from the dead and seated Him at His right hand in the heavenly places, far above all principality and power and might and dominion, and every name that is named, not only in this age but also in that which is to come. And He put all things under His feet, and gave Him to be head over all things to the church," (Ephesians 1:19-22 NKJV)*

"...He will reign over the house of Jacob forever, and of His kingdom there will be no end."(Luke 1:33 NKJV)*

•

Messiah's Kingdom shall be the Kingdom for the Saints:

Old Testament
"Then the kingdom and dominion, And the greatness of the kingdoms under the whole heaven, Shall be given to the people, the saints of the Most High. His kingdom is an everlasting kingdom, And all dominions shall serve and obey Him.'" (Daniel 7:27 NKJV)*

New Testament
"Then comes the end, when He delivers the kingdom to God the Father, when He puts an end to all rule and all authority and power." (1 Corinthians 15:24 NKJV)*

"Then the seventh angel sounded: And there were loud voices in heaven, saying, "The kingdoms of this world have become the kingdoms of our Lord and of His Christ, and He shall reign forever and ever!" (Revelation 11:15 NKJV)*

•

The Messiah shall be anointed, make reconciliation for sins and bring everlasting righteousness:

Old Testament
"Seventy weeks are determined For your people and for your holy city, To finish the transgression, To make an end of sins, To make reconciliation for iniquity, To bring in everlasting righteousness, To seal up vision and prophecy, And to anoint the Most Holy." (Daniel 9:24 NKJV)*

New Testament
"Grace to you and peace from God the Father and our Lord Jesus Christ, who gave Himself for our sins, that He might deliver us from this present evil age, according to the will of our God and Father, to whom be glory forever and ever. Amen." (Galatians 1:3-5 NKJV)*

289

"And the angel answered and said to her, "The Holy Spirit will come upon you, and the power of the Highest will overshadow you; therefore, also, that Holy One who is to be born will be called the Son of God." (Luke 1:35 NKJV)*

•

The Messiah's arrival predicted to the exact day (483 years) from the command to rebuild the city of Jerusalem:

Old Testament

"Know therefore and understand,That from the going forth of the command To restore and build Jerusalem Until Messiah the Prince, There shall be seven weeks and sixty-two weeks; The street shall be built again, and the wall, Even in troublesome times." (Daniel 9:25 NKJV)*

New Testament

"The next day a great multitude that had come to the feast, when they heard that Jesus was coming to Jerusalem, took branches of palm trees and went out to meet Him, and cried out: " Hosanna! ' Blessed is He who comes in the name of the LORD! ' The King of Israel!" (John 12:12 NKJV)*

•

Messiah shall be killed for the sins of the world before the Temple is destroyed by the Romans:

Old Testament

"And after the sixty-two weeks Messiah shall be cut off, but not for Himself; And the people of the prince who is to come Shall destroy the city and the sanctuary. The end of it shall be with a flood, And till the end of the war desolations are determined." (Daniel 9:26NKJV)*

New Testament

Then they crucified Him, and divided His garments, casting lots, that it might be fulfilled which was spoken by the prophet: "They divided My garments among them, And for My clothing they cast lots." (Matthew 27:35 NKJV)*

"But we see Jesus, who was made a little lower than the angels, for the suffering of death crowned with glory and honor, that He, by the grace of God, might taste death for everyone." (Hebrews 2:9 NKJV)*

"And Jesus cried out again with a loud voice, and yielded up His spirit. Then, behold, the veil of the temple was torn in two from top to bottom; and the earth quaked, and the rocks were split," (Matthew 27:50-51 NKJV)*

•

Messiah's glorified appearance:

Old Testament
"I lifted my eyes and looked, and behold, a certain man clothed in linen, whose waist was girded with gold of Uphaz! His body was like beryl, his face like the appearance of lightning, his eyes like torches of fire, his arms and feet like burnished bronze in color, and the sound of his words like the voice of a multitude." (Daniel 10:5-6 NKJV)*

New Testament
"..and in the midst of the seven lampstands One like the Son of Man, clothed with a garment down to the feet and girded about the chest with a golden band. His head and hair were white like wool, as white as snow, and His eyes like a flame of fire; [15] His feet were like fine brass, as if refined in a furnace, and His voice as the sound of many waters; He had in His right hand seven stars, out of His mouth went a sharp two-edged sword, and His countenance was like the sun shining in its strength." (Revelation 1:13-16 NKJV)*

•

The restoration of Israel:

Old Testament
"For the children of Israel shall abide many days without king or prince, without sacrifice or sacred pillar, without ephod or teraphim. Afterward the children of Israel shall return and seek the LORD their God and David their king. They shall fear the LORD and His goodness in the latter days." (Hosea 3:4-5 NKJV)*

New Testament

"For I do not desire, brethren, that you should be ignorant of this mystery, lest you should be wise in your own opinion, that blindness in part has happened to Israel until the fullness of the Gentiles has come in And so all Israel will be saved, as it is written: " The Deliverer will come out of Zion, And He will turn away ungodliness from Jacob; For this is My covenant with them, When I take away their sins." (Romans 11:25-27 NKJV)*

•

The Messiah to return from Egypt:

Old Testament
"When Israel was a child, I loved him, And out of Egypt I called My son." (Hosea 11:1 NKJV)*

"God brings him out of Egypt; He has strength like a wild ox; He shall consume the nations, his enemies; He shall break their bones And pierce them with his arrows." (Numbers 24:8 NKJV)*

New Testament
"When he arose, he took the young Child and His mother by night and departed for Egypt," (Matthew 2:14 NKJV)*

"Now when Herod was dead, behold, an angel of the Lord appeared in a dream to Joseph in Egypt, saying, "Arise, take the young Child and His mother, and go to the land of Israel, for those who sought the young Child's life are dead." Then he arose, took the young Child and His mother, and came into the land of Israel." (Matthew 2:19-21 NKJV)*

•

Messiah to defeat death:

Old Testament
"I will ransom them from the power of the grave; I will redeem them from death. O Death, I will be your plagues! O Grave, I will be your destruction! Pity is hidden from My eyes."" (Hosea 13:14 NKJV)*

New Testament
*"O Death, where is your sting? O Hades, where is your victory? "The sting
of death is sin, and the strength of sin is the law. But thanks be to God,
who gives us the victory through our Lord Jesus Christ." (1 Corinthians
15:55-57 NKJV)**

•

The outpouring of the Spirit:

Old Testament
*" And it shall come to pass afterward That I will pour out My Spirit on all
flesh; Your sons and your daughters shall prophesy, Your old men shall
dream dreams, Your young men shall see visions. And also on My
menservants and on My maidservants I will pour out My Spirit in those
days. "And I will show wonders in the heavens and in the earth: Blood
and fire and pillars of smoke. The sun shall be turned into darkness, And
the moon into blood, Before the coming of the great and awesome day
of the LORD (Judgment Day). And it shall come to pass That whoever
calls on the name of the LORD Shall be saved. For in Mount Zion and in
Jerusalem there shall be deliverance, As the LORD has said, Among the
remnant whom the LORD calls." (Joel 2:28-32 NKJV)**

New Testament
*"And it shall come to pass in the last days, says God, That I will pour out
of My Spirit on all flesh; Your sons and your daughters shall prophesy
Your young men shall see visions, Your old men shall dream dreams.
And on My menservants and on My maidservants I will pour out My
Spirit in those days; And they shall prophesy. I will show wonders in
heaven above And signs in the earth beneath: Blood and fire and vapor
of smoke. The sun shall be turned into darkness, And the moon into
blood, Before the coming of the great and awesome day of the LORD.
And it shall come to pass That whoever calls on the name of the
LORD Shall be saved.' " (Acts 2:17-21 NKJV)**

*For there is no distinction between Jew and Greek, for the same Lord
over all is rich to all who call upon Him. For "whoever calls on the name
of the LORD shall be saved." (Romans 10:12-13 NKJV)**

•

293

Israel shall be regathered:

Old Testament

"I will surely assemble all of you, O Jacob, I will surely gather the remnant of Israel; I will put them together like sheep of the fold, Like a flock in the midst of their pasture; They shall make a loud noise because of so many people. The one who breaks open will come up before them; They will break out, Pass through the gate, And go out by it; Their king will pass before them, With the LORD at their head." (Micah 2:12-13 NKJV)*

New Testament

"I am the good shepherd; and I know My sheep, and am known by My own. As the Father knows Me, even so I know the Father; and I lay down My life for the sheep." (John 10:14 NKJV)*

"My sheep hear My voice, and I know them, and they follow Me. And I give them eternal life, and they shall never perish; neither shall anyone snatch them out of My hand. My Father, who has given them to Me, is greater than all; and no one is able to snatch them out of My Father's hand." (John 10:26 NKJV)*

•

Once Messiah's Kingdom is established He will teach us His ways:

Old Testament

"Many nations shall come and say, " Come, and let us go up to the mountain of the LORD, To the house of the God of Jacob; He will teach us His ways, And we shall walk in His paths." For out of Zion the law shall go forth, And the word of the LORD from Jerusalem. He shall judge between many peoples And rebuke strong nations afar off; They shall beat their swords into plowshares, And their spears into pruning hooks; Nation shall not lift up sword against nation, Neither shall they learn war anymore." (Micah 4:1-8 NKJV)*

New Testament

"And He will reign over the house of Jacob forever, and of His kingdom there will be no end."(Luke 1:33 NKJV)*

"And the nations of those who are saved shall walk in its light, and the kings of the earth bring their glory and honor into it. Its gates shall not be shut at all by day (there shall be no night there). And they shall bring the glory and the honor of the nations into it. But there shall by no means enter it anything that defiles, or causes an abomination or a lie, but only those who are written in the Lamb's Book of Life. (Revelation 21:24-27 NKJV)*

•

The everlasting ruler Messiah to be born in Bethlehem:

Old Testament
"But you, Bethlehem Ephrathah, Though you are little among the thousands of Judah, Yet out of you shall come forth to Me The One to be Ruler in Israel, Whose goings forth are from of old, From everlasting." (Micah 5:2 NKJV)*

New Testament
"Now after Jesus was born in Bethlehem of Judea in the days of Herod the king, behold, wise men from the East came to Jerusalem, saying, "Where is He who has been born King of the Jews? For we have seen His star in the East and have come to worship Him." (Matthew 2:1-2 NKJV)*

Jesus said to them, "Most assuredly, I say to you, before Abraham was, I AM." (John 8:58 NKJV)*

•

The Messiah will visit the second Temple:

Old Testament
"For thus says the LORD of hosts: 'Once more (it is a little while) I will shake heaven and earth, the sea and dry land; and I will shake all nations, and they shall come to the Desire of All Nations, and I will fill this temple with glory,' says the LORD of hosts. 'The silver is Mine, and the gold is Mine,' says the LORD of hosts. 'The glory of this latter temple shall be greater than the former,' says the LORD of hosts. 'And in this place I will give peace,' says the LORD of hosts." (Haggai 2:6-9 NKJV)*

So he came by the Spirit into the temple. And when the parents brought in the Child Jesus, to do for Him according to the custom of the law, he took Him up in his arms and blessed God and said: " Lord, now You are letting Your servant depart in peace, According to Your word; For my eyes have seen Your salvation Which You have prepared before the face of all peoples, A light to bring revelation to the Gentiles, And the glory of Your people Israel." (Luke2:27-32 NKJV)*

•

Messiah a descendant of Zerubabel:

Old Testament
'In that day,' says the LORD of hosts, 'I will take you, Zerubbabel My servant, the son of Shealtiel,' says the LORD, 'and will make you like a signet ring; for I have chosen you,' says the LORD of hosts." (Haggai 2:23 NKJV)*

New Testament
"Now Jesus Himself began His ministry at about thirty years of age, being (as was supposed) the son of Joseph, the son of Heli, the son of Matthat, the son of Levi, the son of Melchi, the son of Janna, the son of Joseph, the son of Mattathiah, the son of Amos, the son of Nahum, the son of Esli, the son of Naggai, the son of Maath, the son of Mattathiah, the son of Semei, the son of Joseph, the son of Judah, the son of Joannas, the son of Rhesa, the son of Zerubbabel, the son of Shealtiel, the son of Neri," (Luke 3:23-27 NKJV)*

•

Earthquake and the Sun darkened at Messiah's humilation and death:

Old Testament
"Shall the land not tremble for this, And everyone mourn who dwells in it? All of it shall swell like the River, Heave and subside Like the River of Egypt. " And it shall come to pass in that day," says the Lord GOD, " That I will make the sun go down at noon, And I will darken the earth in broad daylight; I will turn your feasts into mourning, And all your songs into lamentation; I will bring sackcloth on every waist, And baldness on

every head; I will make it like mourning for an only son, And its end like a bitter day." (Amos 8:8-10 NKJV)*

New Testament

"Now from the sixth hour until the ninth hour there was darkness over all the land. And about the ninth hour Jesus cried out with a loud voice, saying, "Eli, Eli, lama sabachthani?" that is, "My God, My God, why have You forsaken Me?" Some of those who stood there, when they heard that, said, "This Man is calling for Elijah!" Immediately one of them ran and took a sponge, filled it with sour wine and put it on a reed, and offered it to Him to drink. The rest said, "Let Him alone; let us see if Elijah will come to save Him."And Jesus cried out again with a loud voice, and yielded up His spirit. Then, behold, the veil of the temple was torn in two from top to bottom; and the earth quaked, and the rocks were split," (Matthew 27:45-51 NKJV)*

•

Messiah is the high Priest and King:

Old Testament

"Then speak to him, saying, 'Thus says the LORD of hosts, saying: " Behold, the Man whose name is the BRANCH! From His place He shall branch out, And He shall build the temple of the LORD; Yes, He shall build the temple of the LORD. He shall bear the glory, And shall sit and rule on His throne; So He shall be a priest on His throne, And the counsel of peace shall be between them both.'" (Zechariah 6:12-13 NKJV)*

New Testament

"Now this is the main point of the things we are saying: We have such a High Priest, who is seated at the right hand of the throne of the Majesty in the heavens," (Hebrews 8:1 NKJV)*

•

The old covenant is broken; God's protection is taken away:

Old Testament

"Thus says the LORD my God, "Feed the flock for slaughter, whose owners slaughter them and feel no guilt; those who sell them say,

'Blessed be the LORD, for I am rich'; and their shepherds do not pity them. For I will no longer pity the inhabitants of the land," says the LORD. "But indeed I will give everyone into his neighbor's hand and into the hand of his king. They shall attack the land, and I will not deliver them from their hand." So I fed the flock for slaughter, in particular the poor of the flock. I took for myself two staffs: the one I called Beauty, and the other I called Bonds; and I fed the flock. I dismissed the three shepherds in one month. My soul loathed them, and their soul also abhorred me. Then I said, "I will not feed you. Let what is dying die, and what is perishing perish. Let those that are left eat each other's flesh." And I took my staff, Beauty, and cut it in two, that I might break the covenant which I had made with all the peoples. So it was broken on that day. Thus the poor of the flock, who were watching me, knew that it was the word of the LORD." (Zachariah 11:4-11 NKJV)*

New Testament
"Now as He drew near, He saw the city and wept over it, saying, "If you had known, even you, especially in this your day, the things that make for your peace! But now they are hidden from your eyes. For days will come upon you when your enemies will build an embankment around you, surround you and close you in on every side, and level you, and your children within you, to the ground; and they will not leave in you one stone upon another, because you did not know the time of your visitation." (Luke 19:41-44 NKJV)*

"For this is My blood of the new covenant, which is shed for many for the remission of sins." (Matthew 26:28 NKJV)*

•

Messiah betrayed for thirty pieces of silver:

Old Testament
"Then I said to them, "If it is agreeable to you, give me my wages; and if not, refrain." So they weighed out for my wages thirty pieces of silver. And the LORD said to me, "Throw it to the potter"—that princely price they set on me. So I took the thirty pieces of silver and threw them into the house of the LORD for the potter." (Zachariah 11:12-13 NKJV)*

"Then one of the twelve, called Judas Iscariot, went to the chief priests and said, "What are you willing to give me if I deliver Him to you?" And they counted out to him thirty pieces of silver." (Matthew 26:14-15 NKJV)*

"Then Judas, His betrayer, seeing that He had been condemned, was remorseful and brought back the thirty pieces of silver to the chief priests and elders, saying, "I have sinned by betraying innocent blood." And they said, "What is that to us? You see to it!" Then he threw down the pieces of silver in the temple and departed, and went and hanged himself. But the chief priests took the silver pieces and said, "It is not lawful to put them into the treasury, because they are the price of blood." And they consulted together and bought with them the potter's field, to bury strangers in. Therefore that field has been called the Field of Blood to this day. Then was fulfilled what was spoken by Jeremiah the prophet, saying, "And they took the thirty pieces of silver, the value of Him who was priced, whom they of the children of Israel priced, and gave them for the potter's field, as the LORD directed me." (Matthew 27:3-10 NKJV)*

•

The Messiah would be pierced:

Old Testament
"And I will pour on the house of David and on the inhabitants of Jerusalem the Spirit of grace and supplication; then they will look on Me whom they pierced. Yes, they will mourn for Him as one mourns for his only son, and grieve for Him as one grieves for a firstborn." (Zachariah 12:10 NKJV)*

New Testament
"But one of the soldiers pierced His side with a spear, and immediately blood and water came out." (John 19:34 NKJV)*

•

The Messiah will be killed and the flock scattered, the nation's protection taken away and the nation scattered:

Old Testament
"Awake, O sword, against My Shepherd, Against the Man who is My Companion," Says the LORD of hosts. "Strike the Shepherd, And the

sheep will be scattered; Then I will turn My hand against the little ones."
(Zachariah 13:7 NKJV)*

New Testament
"Then they crucified Him, and divided His garments, casting lots, that it might be fulfilled which was spoken by the prophet: "They divided My garments among them, And for My clothing they cast lots." (Matthew 27:35 NKJV)*

"In that hour Jesus said to the multitudes, "Have you come out, as against a robber, with swords and clubs to take Me? I sat daily with you, teaching in the temple, and you did not seize Me. But all this was done that the Scriptures of the prophets might be fulfilled." Then all the disciples forsook Him and fled." (Matthew 26:55-56 NKJV)*

•

A messenger will prepare the way for the Messiah, messenger of the new covenant:

Old Testament
"Behold, I send My messenger, And he will prepare the way before Me. And the Lord, whom you seek, Will suddenly come to His temple, Even the Messenger of the covenant, In whom you delight. Behold, He is coming," Says the LORD of hosts." (Malachi 3:1 NKJV)*

New Testament
"For this is he of whom it is written: 'Behold, I send My messenger before Your face, Who will prepare Your way before You." (Matthew 11:10 NKJV)*

"And for this reason He is the Mediator of the new covenant, by means of death, for the redemption of the transgressions under the first covenant, that those who are called may receive the promise of the eternal inheritance." (Hebrews 9:15 NKJV)*

Recommended Reading

Mysteries of the Kingdom Revealed
By Luis E. Caquias
INFINITY PUBLISHING
1094 New DeHaven Street, Suite 100
West Conshohocken, PA 19428-2713

Jesus in the Feasts of Israel
By Richard Booker
BRIDGE PUBLISHING, INC.
South Plainfield, New Jersey

JESUS Among Other Gods
By Ravi Zacharias
Published by Word Publishing
Nashville, Tenn.
Thomas Nelson Company

Creation Triumphs Over Evolution
Published by Bible Students Congregation
of New Brunswick
PO Box 144
Edison NJ 08818-0144 bible411.com

Endnotes

[1] Clark, Ronald W. *Einstein: A Life and Times.* The World Publishing Company, 1971, p. 99.

[2] Michael Behe, DARWIN'S BLACK BOX (New York: The Free Press, 1996), 39. Darwin, C.,The Origin of Species, 6th ed (1988), NYU Press, NY, 154.

[3] Clyde A. Hutchinson, III et al., "Global Transposon Mutagenesis and a Minimal Mycoplasma Genome," *Science* 286 (1999), 2165-69.

[4] Nikos Kyrpides et al., "Universal Protein Families and the Functional Content of the Last Universal Common Ancestor," *Journal of Molecular Evolution* 49 (1999): 413-23.

[5] Hubert Yockey, INFORMATION THEORY AND MOLECULAR BIOLOGY (New York: Cambridge University, 1992), 198, 246-257.

[6] Richard Losick and Lucy Shapiro, "Changing Views on the Nature of the Bacterial Cell: From Biochemistry to Cytology," *Journal of Bacteriology* 181(1999): 4143-45.

[7] Creation Triumphs Over Evolution, Published by: Bible Students Congregation of New Brunswick PO Box 144 Edison NJ 08818-0144 bible411.com chap. Vpg 30-52

[8] Robert L. Dorit, Hiroshi Akashi and Walter Gilbert, "Absence of Polymorphism at the ZFY Locus on the Human Y Chromosome," *Science,* 268 (1995), 1183-1185; Svante Paabo, "The Y Chromosome and the Origin of All of US (Men)," *Science,* 268 (1995), 1141-1142.

[9] Molecular History Research Center, www.mhr.net/mitochondrialEve.htm 8-10-2010

[10] Wes Burrows and Oliver A. Ryder, "Y-Chromosome Variation in Great Apes," Nature, 385 (1997), pp. 125-126.

[11] Panin, Ivan. *Verbal Inspiration of the Bible Scientifically Demonstrated.* Toronto, Canada: Armach Press, 1923.

[12] Brooks, Keith L., Ph.D. *Absolute Mathematical Proofs of the Divine Inspiration of the Bible, Comments on the Works of Panin.* 7600 Jubilee Drive, Niagara Falls, Ontario, Canada L2G 7J6: Bible Numerics.

[13] Ibid.

[14] Booker, Richard. *Jesus in the Feasts of Israel.* South Plainfield, New Jersey: Bridge Publishing, Inc., 1987, pp. 17–25.

[15] Zacharias, Ravi. *JESUS Among Other Gods.* Nashville, Tennessee: Word Publishing, A Thomas Nelson Company, 2000, pp. 40–42.

[16] Tabor, James D., Ph.D. *The Jewish Roman World of Jesus.* "Josephus, Antiquities," 1998, 18.63–64.

[17] Ibid.

[18] Eisenman, Robert. *James the Brother of Jesus.* Viking Penguin, a division of Penguin Books USA, Inc., 1997, pp. 289–291.

[19] http://www.creationmoments.com/articles/article.php?a=208&c=4/11-28-09.

[20] Lead Toxicity: Who Is at Risk of Lead Exposure?". United States Center for Disease Control: Agency for Toxic Substances and Disease Registry. http://www.atsdr.cdc.gov/csem/lead/pbwhoisat_risk2.html. 8-25-2009.

PRAYER OF SALVATION

Father Yahveh,
My God and Creator;
Forgive me Father for sinning against You, and
for not making you the priority of my life.
Thank You for sacrificing Your Son to restore me to You.
I accept Yahshua as my Lord and Savior.
Help me to change to be like Yahshua;
That His Spirit dwell in me and guide me.
Help me to be an example to others;
As Yahshua was an example to me.
I pray that salvation come to my family and friends.
That I may serve and glorify You in all that I do.
In the name above all names I ask you Father;
Yahshua my Messiah and King.

Amen

Questions, Contact and Comments:

theIdealbodybook Club
Purchase signed books

www.theidealbodybook.com

CPSIA information can be obtained at www.ICGtesting.com
Printed in the USA
LVOW11s2327150114

369640LV00014B/559/P